Minimally Invasive Surgery in Orthopedics

T0210434

Giles R. Scuderi • Alfred J. Tria

Editors

Minimally Invasive Surgery in Orthopedics

Upper Extremity Handbook

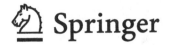 Springer

Editors
Giles R. Scuderi
Insall Scott Kelly Institute
New York, USA
grscuderi@aol.com

Alfred J. Tria
Orthopaedic Center of New Jersey
Somerset New Jersey
Suite 1300, USA
atriajrmd@aol.com

ISBN 978-1-4614-0672-3   e-ISBN 978-1-4614-0673-0
DOI 10.1007/978-1-4614-0673-0
Springer New York Dordrecht Heidelberg London

Library of Congress Control Number: 2011936131

Printed on acid-free paper

Springer is part of Springer Science+Business Media (www.springer.com)

Contents

Contributors

Kenneth Accousti, MD Shoulder Fellow,
Mount Sinai Medical Center, New York, NY, USA

David W. Altchek, MD Professor, Department of Orthopaedic Surgery,
Weill Medical College of Cornell University, New York, NY, USA
Co-Chief, Sports Medicine and Shoulder Service,
Hospital for Special Surgery, New York, NY, USA

John-Erik Bell, MD Assistant Professor, Shoulder, Elbow and Sports
Medicine, Department of Orthopaedic Surgery, Dartmouth-Hitchcock
Medical Center, Lebanon, NH, USA

Louis U. Bigliani, MD Frank E. Stinchfield Professor and Chairman,
Department of Orthopaedic Surgery, New York-Presbyterian Hospital,
Columbia University Medical Center, New York, NY, USA

Theodore A. Blaine, MD Associate Professor, Department of Orthopaedic
Surgery, Brown Alpert Medical School, Providence, RI, USA
Rhode Island Hospital and the Miriam Hospitals, Providence, RI, USA

Louis W. Catalano III, MD Assistant Clinical Professor,
Department of Orthopaedic Surgery, Columbia College of Physicians
and Surgeons, New York, NY, USA
Attending Hand Surgeon, C.V. Starr Hand Surgery Center,
St. Luke's-Roosevelt Hospital Center, New York, NY, USA

Frances Cuomo, MD Chief, Division of Shoulder and Elbow Surgery,
Department of Orthopedics and Sports Medicine, Beth Israel
Medical Center, Philips Ambulatory Care Center, New York, NY, USA

Phani K. Dantuluri, MD Assistant Clinical Professor,
Department of Orthopaedics, Thomas Jefferson University Hospital,
Jefferson Medical College, The Philadelphia Hand Center,
Philadelphia, PA, USA

Christopher C. Dodson, MD Fellow, Sports Medicine
and Shoulder Service, Hospital for Special Surgery, New York, NY, USA

Xavier Duralde, MD Private Practice, Peachtree Orthopaedic Clinic, Atlanta, GA, USA

Sara L. Edwards, MD Fellow, Department of Orthopedic Surgery, New York-Presbyterian Hospital, Columbia University Medical Center, New York, NY, USA

Evan L. Flatow, MD Lasker Professor and Chair, Peter & Leni May Department of Orthopaedic Surgery, Mount Sinai Medical Center, New York, NY, USA

W. Anthony Frisella, MD, MA Fellow, Shoulder and Elbow Service Department of Orthopedics and Sports Medicine, Beth Israel Medical Center, Philips Ambulatory Care Center, New York, NY, USA

Leesa M. Galatz, MD Associate Professor, Program Director, Should & Elbow Fellowship, Department of Orthopaedic Surgery, Washington University School of Medicine, St. Louis, MO, USA

Steven Z. Glickel, MD Associate Clinical Professor of Orthopaedic Surgery, Columbia College of Physicians and Surgeons, New York, NY, USA

Director, Hand Service, C.V. Starr Hand Surgery Center, St. Luke's-Roosevelt Hospital Center, New York, NY, USA

Michael R. Hausman, MD Professor, Department of Orthopaedics, Mount Sinai School of Medicine, New York, NY, USA

Jonathon Herald, MD Department of Orthopaedics, Mount Sinai School of Medicine, New York, NY, USA

Jim C. Hsu, MD Private Practice, The Sports Medicine Clinic, Seattle, WA, USA

Raymond A. Klug, MD Assistant Professor, Department of Orthopaedics, Mount Sinai School of Medicine, New York, NY, USA

Edward W. Lee, MD Attending Surgeon, The CORE Institute, Phoenix, AZ, USA

Steve K. Lee, MD Associate Chief, Division of Hand Surgery, Department of Orthopaedic Surgery, The NYU Hospital for Joint Diseases, New York, NY, USA

Assistant Professor, Department of Orthopaedic Surgery, The New York University School of Medicine, New York, NY, USA

Co-Chief, Hand Surgery Service, Bellevue Hospital Center, New York, NY, USA

Brian Magovern, MD Attending Physician, Shoulder Service, Harbor-UCLA Medical Center, Private Practice, Orthopaedic Institute, Torrance, CA, USA

Guido Marra, MD Assistant Professor, Chief, Section of Shoulder and Elbow Surgery, Loyola University medical Center, Maywood, IL, USA

Bradford O. Parsons, MD Assistant Professor, Department
of Orthopaedics, Mount Sinai School of Medicine, New York, NY, USA

Milan M. Patel, MD Fellow, C.V. Starr Hand Surgery Center,
St. Luke's-Roosevelt Hospital Center, New York, NY, USA

Matthew L. Ramsey, MD Private Practice, Rothman Institute,
Philadelphia, PA, USA

Aaron G. Rosenberg, MD Professor, Department of Orthopaedic Surgery,
Rush Medical College, Rush-Presbyterian-St. Luke's Center,
Chicago, IL, USA

Steven J. Thornton, MD Fellow, Department of Orthopaedic Surgery,
Hospital for Special Surgery, New York, NY, USA

Mordechai Vigler, MD Chief of Hand Surgery, Department
of Orthopaedic Surgery, Rabin Medical Center, Hasharon Hospital,
Tel-Aviv University, Sackler School of Medicine, Petach-Tikva, Israel

What Is Minimally Invasive Surgery and How Do You Learn It?

Aaron G. Rosenberg

Innovation in surgery is not new and should not be unexpected. As an example, the history of total joint replacement has demonstrated continuous evolution, and the relatively high complication rates associated with early prostheses and techniques eventually led to the improvement of implants and refinement of the surgical procedures. Gradual adoption of these improvements and their eventual diffusion into the surgical community led to improved success and increased rates of implantation [1]. Increased surgical experience was eventually accompanied by more rapid surgical performance and then by the development of standardized hospitalization protocols, which eventually led to more rapid rehabilitation and return to function. These benefits are well accepted and can be seen as helping contribute to the establishment of a more "consumer driven" and medical practice.

Most surgeons would agree that as experience guides the surgeon to more accurate incision placement, more precise dissection, and more skillful mobilization of structure, the need for *wide* exposure diminishes. Indeed, less invasiveness appears to be a hallmark of experience gained with a given procedure. From a historical perspective, this appears to be true of total hip replacement. The operation as initially described by Charnley required trochanteric osteotomy. The osteotomy served several purposes: generous exposure, access to the intramedullary canal for proper component placement and cement pressurization, and the ability of the surgeon to "tension" the abductors to improve stability. However, over time, it became apparent that trochanteric nonunion and retained trochanteric hardware could be problematic. In attempts to minimize these problems, some worked to develop improved techniques for trochanteric fixation. However, others went in a different direction, eventually demonstrating that the operation could be performed quite adequately without osteotomy. Many purists complained that this was not the Charnley operation, and that the *benefits* of trochanteric osteotomy were lost. Yet the eventual acceptance of the nonosteotomy approaches by almost all surgeons performing primary total hip arthroplasty (THA) in the vast majority of circumstances would attest to the fact that osteotomy was not required to achieve the result that had come to be expected.

These developments led to the popularity of the posterior approach to the hip for THA. Initially the gluteus maximus tendon insertion into the postero-lateral femur was routinely taken down to obtain adequate exposure of the acetabulum. Indeed, the generous exposure provided by this release was needed to adequately control acetabular component position, to reduce bleeding for cement interdigitation, and to allow pressurization of acetabular cement. However, this generous exposure was associated with a higher dislocation rate than was

A.G. Rosenberg (✉)
Department of Orthopaedic Surgery,
Rush Medical College, Rush-Presbyterian-St. Luke's
Center, Chicago, IL, USA

G.R. Scuderi and A.J. Tria (eds.), *Minimally Invasive Surgery in Orthopedics: Upper Extremity Handbook*,
DOI 10.1007/978-1-4614-0673-0_1, © Springer Science+Business Media, LLC 2012

seen with the trochanteric osteotomy technique. But with the advent of improved component design (offset) and better understanding of component positioning, as well as the introduction of cementless techniques, less exposure was needed in the majority of cases. Eventually, careful closure of the posterior structures also led to a significant reduction in the dislocation rate [2]. Seen in this example is a finding typically noted in the close examination of most evolutionary processes: initial benefits are obtained at some expense in the form of new or different complications or alterations in the complication rate. Further modifications are then required to overcome the new problems that arise from the adaptation of the innovation. The study of the factors that lead to the adoption (and alterations) of innovations has been extensively studied by Rogers and is well described in his landmark work, *The Diffusion of Innovation* [3].

The trend to *less* or minimally invasive procedures has been noted in other specialties [4] and perhaps can be seen most dramatically in the field of interventional radiology [5].

It would be fair to say that almost all surgical techniques improve over time by leading to less invasive approaches, which are frequently adopted only reluctantly by the surgical community. For skeptics it is instructive to review the career of Dr. Kurt Semm [6]. His reports of surgical techniques were shouted down at professional meetings and his lectures were greeted with "laughter, derision, and suspicion." He was forbidden to publish by his dean, and his first papers submitted were rejected because they were "unethical." The President of the German Surgical Society demanded that his license be revoked and he be barred from practice. His associates at the University of Kiel asked him to have psychological testing because his ideas were considered so radical. Despite this opprobrium, he invented 80 patented surgical devices, published more than 1,000 scientific papers, and developed dozens of new techniques. His obituary in the *The British Medical Journal* hailed him as "the father of laparoscopic surgery." Who today would choose a standard open cholecystectomy over the benefits of the laparoscopic approach?

Hip replacement is currently being performed by a variety of minimalist modifications of the standard hip approaches as well as by nontraditional approaches. Knee replacement is similarly being attempted through shorter incisions with various arthrotomy approaches. The proponents of all call them *minimally invasive*, but this term has really become a catchall, and has no specificity or agreed upon meaning.

The purported benefits of these techniques include earlier, more rapid, and more complete recovery of function, less perioperative bleeding, and improved cosmesis. There has been, to date, few data by other than those proponents of specific techniques to substantiate any of these potential benefits. Of course, these purported benefits must be weighed against their potential to change the nature and/or incidence of complications that may arise secondary to the modifications of these approaches.

There is general consensus that adoption of new techniques initially results in a greater incidence of complications. This is the so-called learning curve [7, 8], well known to all surgeons learning a new procedure. Whether this learning curve is extended or contracted has been shown to depend on both individual as well as the systemic features of the operation [9].

It should therefore come as little surprise that, in the hands of those initially reporting these modified procedures (and presumably who have developed their expertise gradually and over considerable time), the complication rates are comparable to those found in the standard approaches, while others report a higher complication rate [10–14]. There has been insufficient time for the scientific evidence to accumulate in sufficient volume to clarify the specific benefits and risks of these modifications in the hands of specialist surgeons, let alone the generalist who performs these procedures.

Clearly, the modern era's communications technologies, coupled with more sophisticated marketing techniques, have dramatically influenced the speed with which new techniques are recognized, popularized, and thus demanded by an easily influenced public. However, continued accumulation of data through the performance of appropriate studies will eventually determine the most appropriate role for these techniques in the orthopedic surgeon's armamentarium [15]. Prior to that occurrence, what is the surgeon to do?

A purely prescriptive approach is prohibited by the multifactorial nature of the surgical endeavor. The vast majority of surgeons who perform THA on a regular basis have already modified their operative approaches to incorporate less invasive techniques. Each surgeon has an individual tolerance for and willingness to undergo the struggles involved in learning a new procedure, differing levels of commitment to the change required for the performance of the technique, as well as a varying ability to tolerate the potential complications encountered while on the so-called learning curve. Unfortunately, the removal of standard visual, auditory, and tactile feedback cues during the performance of these "less" invasive procedures may require the development of alternate cues, which may not be readily available, well established, or assimilated [11]. Thus, the overall complication rate may rise while familiarization with these cues (and the appropriate response to them) matures or while alternate methods of incorporating similar or comparable information is developed. As attempts are made to limit the invasiveness of surgical procedures, surgeons must be prepared to cultivate and take advantage of nontraditional sensory feedback and other alternate visualization methods to direct their efforts. As these evolve, it can be expected that surgical intervention will continue to become less invasive.

The ultimate question implied in the title of this chapter, that is, how to learn a minimally invasive surgery (MIS) technique, can only be answered by first understanding the current methods of surgical training and their relationship to the practice requirements of standard orthopedic procedures. Only then can we evaluate the way these methods relate specifically to the requirements of MIS and so answer the question: do the specific surgical requirements of the MIS procedure require an alteration in the manner in which we train surgeons? An additional implied assumption is the

perception, which appears to be correct but has not yet been rigorously established, that the performance of minimally invasive procedures in the training environment substantially alters the educational experience for the learning surgeon. A series of linked questions is raised that deserves inquiry: (1) What are the performance requirements for MIS surgery? (2) Do they differ substantially from that of routine non-MIS surgery (begging the question of whether we really understand these!)? (3) What are the relationships between surgical training methods and patient outcomes and do we understand these relationships sufficiently well to proceed to alter them in a meaningful fashion? (4) Does the routine adoption of MIS surgical procedures alter the current teaching environment in a way that is deleterious to the learning surgeon? (5) To what extent do the answers to the proceeding questions demand the development of new methods for surgical teaching as regards the MIS procedures? And, finally, (6) What form might this take?

The old adage "It takes 1 year to teach someone how to operate, 5 years to teach them when to operate, and a lifetime to learn when not to operate." seems to make the point that, in the surgeon's repertoire, it is the psychomotor skills that are the easiest and most readily taught. The implication is that the psychomotor skills required in the operating room are substantively different (and easier to teach) than the cognitive skills required. But this is clearly simplistic. Surgical performance is based on a continuous feedback loop of psychomotor performance intimately coupled with cognitive function. It is the continuous and ongoing making of decisions (albeit almost always at a subconscious level for the experienced) in the midst of physical performance that influences the quality of the surgical intervention.

To what extent the development of these cognitive and motor skills, and their interaction, governs the eventual outcome is a complex problem that has not yet been fully investigated and remains poorly understood. It has been said, "Many more surgeons have done a video analysis of their golf swing than have evaluated their operative performance." While there are few studies that have effectively evaluated real-time surgical performance characteristics in a meaningful way, even more fundamentally and unfortunately, there is little research in the realm of surgical education that would help us determine the specific performance requirements for most surgical procedures in general and of less invasive procedures in particular. Additionally, there are few data on the pedagogical aspects of surgical procedure training for either minimally or maximally invasive procedures. A recent comprehensive review of expert performance indicates that there has been more attention directed to the study of musicians, athletes, pilots, and military commanders than to surgeons [16]. Clearly, however, advances in surgical technology and technique has led to a renewed interest in these issues.

While the performance of arthroscopic procedures has resulted in a premium on specific three-dimensional spaciovisualization and psychomotor applications [17, 18], the same is not necessarily true for MIS-type joint replacement procedures. The simple answer to the question regarding the performance skills requirements for MIS surgery is that they are basically those that are found in standard surgical procedures but taken to a higher level. This arises from specific conditions that appear to be inherent in MIS surgery [19].

1. In some respects, the ability to "protect" structures in the standard fashion may be altered in specific ways unique to the surgical procedure, and this may result in a directly proportional decrease in the margin of error for various intraoperative maneuvers.
2. Small errors during the course of the operation may be less easily recognized, and adjusted for, as the procedure progresses, and the implications of these small errors are potentially magnified.
3. Specific anatomic features that increase the degree of difficulty encountered in the performance of a more "open procedure" (stiffness, deformity, poor tissue quality) may be magnified when the procedure is performed in a minimally invasive fashion.
4. Finally, and perhaps most importantly, the development of minimally invasive techniques frequently involves the removal or diminution

of traditional feedback signals that surgeons normally use and have come to rely upon to make continuous adjustments to their performance. Thus, skills that are little needed, infrequently utilized, or have not been previously recognized become of greater consequence. Indeed the loss of standard cues may need to be compensated for in technique-specific ways. Ironically, in the hands of the more experienced surgeon, many of these feedback signals are no longer "conscious," having been assimilated into almost automatic motor responses; this can make the relearning process required more difficult.

Training surgeons to perform these more difficult techniques, with both less room for error and with a different set of feedback signals, would therefore seem to require the development of both traditional surgical skills as well as new ones in ways that guarantee a more demanding performance level than has traditionally been required.

The questioned need for new training methods implies two separate factors that may be driving this concern. First, are current training methods adequate to the task as currently envisioned? Second, does the conversion in the training environment from standard open to MIS procedures degrade the training experience? The answers can be found by evaluating the features of MIS procedures already noted:

1. Visibility of the surgical field is reduced, compromising visual feedback not only to the performing surgeon, but also to the learning surgeon dependent upon observation and demonstration of anatomy and surgical pathology.
2. Lowered margins for error limit the opportunities awarded to the less experienced trainee; while
3. The decreased ability of the instructor to monitor trainee performance degrades the learning environment.
4. The alteration of traditional cues and their replacement with more subtle and poorly defined feedback signals are hallmarks of MIS techniques. Thus, the replacement of standard open surgery by the MIS procedure would appear to significantly alter the training environment.

Are the traditional residency education and continuing medical education (CME) surgical training methods capable of meeting this standard? The system as currently constituted is derived (with little improvement and perhaps even development of some newer flaws) from the traditional systems of apprenticeship that began sometime between the Dark Ages and the development of city-states in the Renaissance [20]. In this pedagogical method, adapted by the German surgical schools of Kocher and Billroth, and modified in the United States by Halsted, has changed relatively little over the years. Thus, training methodologies used to teach surgical skills remain relatively primitive and have enjoyed little improvement in either theory or practice over the decades. Yet the specific technical requirements of the surgical procedures increase steadily. The combined requirements of residency education, that is, service and education, frequently seem to serve the best interest of neither. Even worse, depending on the specific setting, current training methods may be applied unevenly and randomly to the resident participants [21]. The common cliché, see one, do one, teach one, seems to summarize the cavalier approach to procedural teaching that has been the mainstay of surgical pedagogy. Moreover, when real patients are used for surgical teaching purposes, increased morbidity, prolonged intervention times, and suboptimal results may be expected [22]. It is clear that future technologies, whether they be traditionally surgical or otherwise procedurally interventional, will require more, rather than less, highly structured training and assessment methods. It has been demonstrated that laparoscopic surgery adapts poorly to the standard apprenticeship models for general surgical training. Rather, standardized skill acquisition and validation, performance goals, and a supervised, enforced, skill-based curriculum that readily can be shared between trainee and instructor are thought to be needed to replace the observation and incremental skill acquisition model used in an open surgical environment [23].

Assuming no dramatic change in the nature of our economy and the emphasis on health care, it is not likely that the drive toward less invasive techniques will abate. As technology matures,

new and improved techniques for vital structure protection, component placement and positioning, and bone and soft tissue management will come on line. As they do, the gradual development of improved skill levels in the performance of standard procedures coupled with the cautious adoption of new practices as these skills mature is warranted. An understanding of the ethical and moral responsibilities of the operating surgeon must be understood as they relate to training and surgical performance [24]. An open mind along with a critical eye will be required. The following suggestions can be offered to the surgeon who has yet to adopt these techniques.

How to Learn MIS: Practical Suggestions

It has been demonstrated that domain-specific and task-specific skills are not necessarily readily transferred to new domains or tasks in the surgical environment [25–27]. Surgeons, like other adults, learn best by doing, by practicing what they do, and by challenging themselves to take on increasingly difficult scenarios. Practice, in order to be effective, requires deconstruction of the actual procedure into key elements, each of which is repeated until optimal results are achieved before moving onto the next element. The key ingredient to successful practice and ultimate self-improvement as a surgeon, as in other pursuits in life, is that one be self-motivated and competitive, with a strong desire to improve coupled with appropriate practice routines that can lead to improvement. This calls to mind the old joke, "Mister, How do I get to Carnegie Hall?" The answer, of course, is "practice."

Incremental Improvement Through Practice

The literature on CME provides no support for the hypothesis that didactic CME improves either practice patterns, skill levels, or patient outcomes – from this, one can infer that surgeons learn the more complex domain of surgical performance through repetition of procedures [28]. Willingness to engage in repetitive attempts at improving the quality of what one is doing is crucial. One needs to define clearly the areas requiring practice and employ a gradual, repetitive practice pattern; ultimately, one either improves or must change practice habits. This is particularly important in developing an action plan for surgeons who may not currently be performing any MIS procedures.

Practice

Correct practice begins with the break down of the procedure into its component parts, focusing performance-based exercise on those component parts, and acquiring and recognizing feedback, both during the performance in real time and after. As an example, surgeons who are the most experienced in total knee replacement arthroplasty (TKA) frequently perform the vast majority of the needed soft tissue releases to balance the knee during the initial approach and exposure of the knee. Less experienced surgeons tend to make the soft tissue releases a separate part of the technique, independent of the exposure, while the more experienced surgeon utilizes feedback throughout the procedure and employs it to guide the degree of tissue they are releasing during the exposure. In order to master the new skills that may be required in minimally invasive approaches, the surgeon must reenter the mind of the learner that was present at an earlier stage of training. The basic steps must be isolated, and renewed attention must be given to the details of procedure used to isolate those parts of the operation that require more attention, and there must be a detailed focus on accomplishing the specific tasks required at each step of the procedure, specifically, on how they present new or different challenges. Those steps that require the acquisition of new or refined skills can then receive the appropriate attention. The use of computer guidance can aggressively strengthen feedback loops for surgical technique that might otherwise take years to develop. The precision of the technology provides objective and exacting criticism.

Criticism

Another contributor to effective practice is self-grading. Over time, one increases the pressure on oneself to perform, grades the result, and seeks to improve. Self-grading requires measurement, and one needs to have some surgical goals in mind, such as tourniquet time, time to complete the procedure, or specific objective characteristics of operative performance; cement mantle quality, component position, limb alignment, etc. For more detail on this technique, see the Debriefing section below.

Varied Pressure

Surgeons can expand or contract the amount of pressure experienced, because these less invasive approaches and the procedures themselves are, for the most part, relatively extensile. Beginning a TKA as an MIS procedure does not lock the surgeon into that pathway; if, at any point, the surgeon deems the case too complex or the soft tissue considerations are becoming unexpectedly difficult, no harm is done by increasing the size of the incision to expand the exposure. Surgeons can literally "push the envelope" by working their way from the larger incision down to the smaller and, as a consequence, gradually increase the pressure on themselves. But the surgeon can also reduce that stress when desired or, more importantly, when necessary to achieve the optimal surgical outcome.

Avoid Multiple Learning Curves

It is essential to avoid combining multiple learning curves when learning a new procedure. The outcome of any surgical intervention is clearly multifactorial. Beyond the limitation of one's own surgical skill set and one's intuition, each operation encompasses a complex set of multiple factors, some of which may remain below the radar screen of the most experienced surgeon.

These factors include, but are not limited to, the relative contributions of our assistants, the characteristics of the specific operating room, and the type of anesthesia being used. Multiple alterations to such a complex system are much more difficult to assimilate than the incremental addition of small changes approached one at a time. For example, it would be less than optimal to try a new technique or a new approach with new instruments, a new implant design, a new scrub technician, and a new surgical assistant all at the same time. Avoiding multiple learning curves is essential in ensuring that the pressure you exert upon yourself represents a systematic increase and not an overload; you can sequentially add more complexity and variation as you get better at what you do.

Visualization

Another important technique that has been well publicized in other areas of psychomotor skill acquisition and performance, but not as well publicized in surgery, is the use of visualization techniques. Great athletes will all admit to using visualization as an important part of their practice regimen. Similarly, most high-performing surgeons will also rehearse the operation, literally in their "mind's eye," before proceeding with the case. Most of us who perform complex surgery have the experience of repeatedly reviewing the steps and sequences in a new operation beforehand, particularly when learning something completely new.

Visualization has been used in sports, musical performance, and in other forms of physical activity, including dance and even acrobatic flying. Acrobatic pilots not only visualize the expected sequence of flight maneuvers in their minds along with the control manipulation needed to achieve them, but also assume the corresponding body postures, as if they are experiencing the forces associated with the acrobatic flight maneuver. This visualization technique combines psychomotor and cognitive skill sets. One can similarly see downhill ski racers mentally rehearsing the race course, accompanied by hand and body motion. In the same way, surgeons using similar visualization might "think through" a particular operation sequentially while imagining the potential problems, structures at risk, and specific goals of the procedure, while actually positioning their hands as if they were grasping a specific instrument for a specific task during a surgical procedure.

Debriefing

Another self-improvement method involves debriefing, a more formal model for self, group, or mentor after-activity assessment [29, 30]. The classic role of debriefing is in the military, where it has been used for generations to train and improve the skills of warriors, particularly pilots. Debriefing or after-action reviews involve the meticulous creation of a specific checklist of the goals of any given performance followed by the ruthless assessment of how those goals were actually met during the performance. Debriefing techniques have applications in teaching residents and fellows as well as in improving one's own performance. Such sessions have an important role in improving performance at the step where you are at as well as in successfully ascending the ladder of surgical complexity [31].

Team Approach – Coaching

The MIS effort generally leads to an appreciation of the importance of teamwork and its impact on surgical outcome. Perfect performance of the operation without appropriate attention given to perioperative factors, such as pain control, rehabilitation, etc., will not yield an optimal result. Similarly, increased coordination between assistants and surgeon is another requisite for the successful performance of this more demanding type of surgical procedure. Thus, a continuous focus on the need for a team approach throughout, from preoperative considerations, to the surgical phase, and continuing through to the postoperative environment, is a key determinant of optimal outcome. Every team needs a coach, and, in most cases, the responsibility will and should rest with the surgeon. What do coaches do? Their primary role is to create a feedback loop; this is done by developing performance expectations, monitoring performance in a critical way, and, finally, providing feedback that leads to improvement and both motivates and empowers team members.

The Future

The characteristics that make up surgical performance include preoperative, intraoperative, and postoperative factors. While the focus on surgical training must be on all three arenas, it is mainly the intraoperative phase, where actual physical skills are required, that is seen by most trainees as being the area where there is the least opportunity to develop experience. Experience is ideally gained in an environment where feedback is immediate and mistakes are tolerated as part of the learning experience. One of the things that have prevented surgeons from acquiring greater levels of skill prior to entering practice or even during practice is the lack of such a practice environment.

The performance of surgery itself is dependent on performing multiple "subroutines," most of which have only been available for the surgeon to experience during the performance of actual surgical procedures and therefore presents the surgeon with no real opportunity to "practice" the psychomotor skills required during the procedure. In addition, there is little in the way of immediate information available to the surgeon during the course of the operation that would allow the surgeon to make the type of adjustments that are based on cause-effects/feedback loops. As noted earlier, even in the performance of physical skills, there are multiple cognitive processes that must function correctly and efficiently to maximize surgical performance.

With modern technology, many of the factors that contribute to surgical performance can be simulated and repeatedly experienced with immediate feedback on the correctness of decisions and behaviors. Development and utilization of this technology would be expected to result in any given surgeon moving more rapidly along the learning curve, allowing the surgeon to perform at a higher level during the actual surgical encounter. Despite the obstacles present to the current employment of actual psychomotor skills simulation, these devices will eventually be part of the surgical training environment. In the coming era of virtual reality environments and surgical training simulators, there is good reason to believe that the coupling of these technologies to assist the surgeon in acquiring both motor and cognitive skills will result in improved surgical performance as well as improved patient outcomes as a result of the clinical encounter.

A current potential model for improving surgical responsiveness and judgment can be obtained by using the interactive video game as a model. Several features of the modern interactive video game make it both compelling and popular. One primary feature is the need for continuous involvement by the participant. Lapses of attention cause failure (or loss to an opponent). This need for continuous vigilance by the participant is structured into the gaming environment. This forcing function of involvement leads to a "flow" experience that has been described as exhilarating and involving, compelling attention and participation.

As has been demonstrated in flight simulators, the same environment, appropriately structured, can be used to improve both cognitive judgments as well as response times. The application of structured learning experiences in this type of environment might be expected to achieve remarkable improvements in information transmission, a primary goal of the educational experience.

Of additional import is the current status of computer-guided and computer-assisted procedures to the surgeon's armamentarium. As these technologies become more widely available, the surgeon will need opportunities to practice in the new environment created by the addition of a computerized guidance interface during surgical performance. Familiarity with the structure and content of guidance information, as well as integration of this information with the traditional inputs acquired during surgery, will be needed to improve the real-time intraoperative judgments and physical performance measures needed to perform surgery. This familiarity can best be accomplished in a highly integrated simulation environment.

In order to structure an environment that would provide for progressive advances in cognitive skills acquisition, several requirements must be met. The first requirement is creation of a knowledge base that will be utilized as the cognitive foundation for the simulation technology. This so-called "content knowledge" currently exists in the mind of the surgeons who currently provide education to trainees as well as in text and technique manuals. Second, the knowledge base must be structured so that it can be represented in an algorithmic format with eventual conversion of these algorithms into the type of appropriate branching chain pathways environment, which can be made accessible and modifiable at the computer interface. Third, multiple supplemental elements must be developed to provide a more challenging and robust learning environment. Fourth, an assessment module with accompanying grading mechanism must be developed to couple the quality and intensity of the learning experience to the performance level and other individual educational needs of the learner. Work on cognitive skills development, as well as visual skills acquisition, can be accomplished with little other than content knowledge coupled to appropriate software and computers. This should be the initial focus of development efforts for several reasons. First, investment need not be particularly large for the development of the cognitive skills applications of this technology. Much of the appropriate software currently exists and is utilized in the video gaming industry to structure and create complex interactive environments where multiple elements combine to provide an ever-changing and stimulating participatory environment. The addition of specific physical skills will follow.

Enhancements that will further improve surgical performance can also be introduced to this environment. Appropriately structured to approximate the real-life decisions and judgments that the surgeon will be called upon to make, the addition of creative elements, such as complication/disaster management, head-to-head or machine-based competition, continuous probing for knowledge deficits, and reinforcing functions used to transmit important supplementary and supporting content, will produce a robust learning environment that will make the educational experience engaging, stimulating, challenging, and fun.

While there have been progressive advancements in surgical technology and techniques over the past century, there is excellent evidence that exponentially increasing rates of technology growth will provide an ever more rapidly growing rate of change in the methods whereby surgery is performed. While manual skill performance is likely to remain a mainstay of the surgeons experience, increasing reliance on machine performance and even intelligence would seem to be likely. The surgeon trained today is not likely to be using technologies similar to those learned during training in the practice environment encountered in 2016. It is incumbent upon the surgeon to maintain an adaptable posture toward acquiring new skills, as well as to maintain and hone current skills in order to prepare for future developments in the field.

References

1. Peltier LF. The history of hip surgery. In: Callaghan JJ, Rosenberg AG, Rubash HE (Eds.). *The Adult Hip.* Lippincott, Philadelphia, 1998, pp. 4–19
2. Dixon MC, Scott RD, Schai PA, Stamos V. A simple capsulorrhaphy in a posterior approach for total hip arthroplasty. J Arthroplasty 2004 19(3):373–6
3. Rogers EM. *The Diffusion of Innovation.* Free Press, New York, 5 edition, 2002
4. Fenton DS, Czervionke LF (Eds.). *Image-Guided Spine Intervention.* W B Saunders, New York, 2002
5. Castaneda-Zuniga WR, Tadavarthy SM, Qia Z. *Interventional Radiology.* Lippincott, Williams & Wilkins, Philadelphia, 3 edition, 1997
6. Tuffs A. Kurt Semm Obituary. Br Med J 2003 (327);397
7. Dincler S, Koller MT, Steurer J, Bachmann LM, Christen D, Buchmann P. Multidimensional analysis of learning curves in laparoscopic sigmoid resection: eight-year results. Dis Colon Rectum 2003 46(10): 1371–8
8. Gallagher AG, Smith CD, Bowers SP, Seymour NE, Pearson A, McNatt S, Hananel D, Satava RM. Psychomotor skills assessment in practicing surgeons experienced in performing advanced laparoscopic procedures. J Am Coll Surg 2003 197(3):479–88
9. McCormick PH, Tanner WA, Keane FB, Tierney S. Minimally invasive techniques in common surgical

procedures: implications for training. Ir J Med Sci 2003 172(1):27–9

10. Berger RA, Duwelius PJ. The two-incision minimally invasive total hip arthroplasty: technique and results. Orthop Clin North Am 2004 35(2):163–72

11. Hartzband, MA. Posterolateral minimal incision for total hip replacement: technique and early results. Orthop Clin North Am 2004 35(2):119–29

12. Howell, JR, Masri, BA, Duncan, CP. Minimally invasive versus standard incision anterolateral hip replacement: a comparative study. Orthop Clin North Am 2004 35(2):153–62

13. Wright JM, Crockett HC, Delgado S, Lyman S, Madsen M, Sculco TP Mini-incision for total hip arthroplasty: a prospective, controlled investigation with 5-year follow-up evaluation. J Arthroplasty 2004 19(5):538–45

14. Woolson ST, Mow CS, Syquia JF, Lannin JV, Schurman DJ. Comparison of primary total hip replacements performed with a standard incision or a mini-incision. J Bone Joint Surg Am 2004 86A(7): 1353–8

15. Callaghan JJ, Crowninshield RD, Greenwald AS, Lieberman JR, Rosenberg AG, Lewallen DG. Symposium: introducing technology into orthopaedic practice. How should it be done? J Bone Joint Surg Am 2005 87(5):1146–58

16. Ericsson KA, Charness N, Feltovich PJ, Hoffman RR. *The Cambridge Handbook of Expertise and Expert Performance.* Cambridge University Press, Cambridge, 2006

17. Wilhelm DM, Ogan K, Roehrborn CG, Cadeddu JA, Pearle MS. Assessment of basic endoscopic performance using a virtual reality simulator. J Urol 2003 170(2 Pt 1):692

18. Gallagher AG, Smith CD, Bowers SP, Seymour NE, Pearson A, McNatt S, Hananel D, Satava RM. Psychomotor skills assessment in practicing surgeons experienced in performing advanced laparoscopic procedures. J Am Coll Surg 2003 197(3):479–88

19. McCormick PH, Tanner WA, Keane FB, Tierney S. Minimally invasive techniques in common surgical procedures: implications for training. Ir J Med Sci 2003 172(1):27–9

20. Amirault RJ, Branson R. Educators and expertise: a brief history of theories and models. In: Ericsson KA, Charness N, Feltovich PJ, Hoffman RR (Eds.). *The Cambridge Handbook of Expertise and Expert Performance.* Cambridge University Press, Cambridge, 2006, pp. 72–4

21. Zhou W, Lin PH, Bush RL, Lumsden AB. Endovascular training of vascular surgeons: have we made progress? Semin Vasc Surg 2006 19(2):122–6

22. Colt HG, Crawford SW, Galbraith O. Virtual reality bronchoscopy simulation. Chest 2001 120:1333–39

23. Rosser JC, Jr, Rosser LE, Savalgi RS. Skill acquisition and assessment for laparoscopic surgery. Arch Surg 1998 133(6):657–61

24. Rogers DA. Ethical and educational considerations in minimally invasive surgery training for practicing surgeons. Semin Laparosc Surg 2002 9(4):206–11

25. Wanzel KR, Hmastra SJ, Anastakis DJ, Matsumoto ED, Cusimano MD. Effect of visuospatial ability on learning of spatially-complex surgical skills. Lancet 2002 38:617–27

26. Naik VN, Matsumoto ED, Houston PL, Hamstra SJ, Yeung RY-M, Mallon JS, Martire TM. Fibreoptic oral tracheal intubation skills: do manipulation skills learned on a simple model transfer into the operating room Anesthesiology 2001 95:343–48

27. Figert PL, Park AE, Witzke DB, Schwartz RW. Transfer of training in acquiring laparoscopic skills. J Am Coll Surg 2001 193(5):533–7

28. Norman G, Eva K, Brooks L, Hamstra S. Expertise in medicine and surgery. In: Ericsson KA, Charness N, Feltovich PJ, Hoffman RR (Eds.). *The Cambridge Handbook of Expertise and Expert Performance.* Cambridge University Press, Cambridge, 2006

29. Bond WF, Deitrick LM, Eberhardt M, Barr GC, Kane BG, Worrilow CC, Arnold DC, Croskerry P. Cognitive versus technical debriefing after simulation training. Acad Emerg Med 2006 13(3):276–83

30. Moorthy K, Munz Y, Adams S, Pandey V, Darzi A. A human factors analysis of technical and team skills among surgical trainees during procedural simulations in a simulated operating theatre. Ann Surg 2005 242(5):631–9

31. http://www.msr.org.il/R_D/Debriefing_Techniques/

Overview of Shoulder Approaches: Choosing Between Mini-incision and Arthroscopic Techniques

Raymond A. Klug, Bradford O. Parsons, and Evan L. Flatow

In recent years, there has been great interest in minimally invasive orthopedic surgery. Several branches of orthopedics have embraced the principles of minimally invasive surgery, including traumatology [1–3], spinal surgery [4], and adult reconstruction [5–7]. By far the greatest influence has been felt in the field of sports medicine with the introduction, routine, and later obligate use of the arthroscope. Indeed, the days of the open menisectomy or extraarticular anterior cruciate ligament (ACL) reconstruction are almost beyond us, as in these and many other cases, arthroscopic and arthroscopically assisted techniques have become the standard of care. More recently, the field of shoulder and elbow surgery has begun a similar transition; however, a single, distinct difference exists. Previously in sports medicine, the arthroscope was a new tool and standard open procedures were subsequently approached arthroscopically; however, we are currently witnessing a surge of interest in minimally invasive approaches to techniques that are not amenable to arthroscopic treatment, such as arthroplasty [5–7] or plate osteosynthesis for fractures [1–3]. This creates an interesting dilemma: when to choose arthroscopy versus minimally invasive open surgery or even more traditional open approaches.

When to Choose Arthroscopy over Other Approaches

Three key questions must be answered in order to address the above question. First, does some part of the procedure require an open incision? The most obvious example of this is arthroplasty. Because placement of the implant requires an incision at least as large as the implant itself, an open approach cannot be avoided [8]. As described in the subsequent chapters, this incision can be minimized in many cases to just that necessary for placement of the implant, but, regardless, an open approach is still required.

Second, can the necessary exposure be achieved through arthroscopic, arthroscopically assisted, percutaneous, or even mini-open approaches? If adequate exposure cannot be achieved, then conversion to an open technique is required. In many cases, this can be minimized, if not completely avoided, but it must be emphasized that the surgical result must not be compromised by an attempt at minimizing the incision. An example of this is the use of a "reduction portal" for percutaneous pinning of valgus-impacted four-part proximal humerus fractures [9]. In the hands of a skilled surgeon, the utilization of this additional "portal" can obviate the need for open surgery.

Third, can an equivalent or reasonable outcome be achieved with minimally invasive approaches when compared with the more traditional open approach? The obvious example of this, although still debated, is recurrent instability in the contact

R.A. Klug (✉)
Department of Orthopaedics, Mount Sinai School of Medicine, New York, NY, USA

G.R. Scuderi and A.J. Tria (eds.), *Minimally Invasive Surgery in Orthopedics: Upper Extremity Handbook*,
DOI 10.1007/978-1-4614-0673-0_2, © Springer Science+Business Media, LLC 2012

athlete [10]. While open stabilization procedures have been the gold standard, many authorities in the field disagree with this. At the 2006 annual meeting of American Association of Orthopaedic Surgeons (AAOS), an expert panel was assembled to address shoulder disorders in the contact athlete. When asked about open versus arthroscopic treatment of recurrent instability in contact athletes, 100% of the panel remarked that their preferred treatment would be arthroscopic [11].

The Trend Toward Arthroscopy

It is clear that the trend toward arthroscopic techniques is being embraced by the orthopedic community and is not simply the hype created by a small group of arthroscopists trying to push their trade onto the remainder of the orthopedic public. In a 2003 survey of 908 members of the Arthroscopy Association of North America (AANA) and the American Orthopaedic Society for Sports Medicine (AOSSM), the 700 respondents reported that 24% routinely performed rotator cuff repair through an all-arthroscopic approach, compared with only 5% 5 years earlier. At the 2005 AAOS annual meeting, 167 attendees in a symposium on the rotator cuff were asked how they would repair a mobile, 3-cm rotator cuff tear. Sixty-two percent responded that they would repair it using all arthroscopic techniques [12]. This movement toward less invasive surgical approaches does not only apply to arthroscopy, but rather to minimally invasive open approaches as well.

The concept of pure "open" versus "mini-open" or even "arthroscopic" surgery is not well defined. Is an ACL reconstruction with a local patella tendon harvest considered "arthroscopic" if an open approach is used to harvest the graft? What if hamstring tendons are used through a separate incision? Does this make the ACL reconstruction arthroscopic, but the graft harvest open? Or mini-open? What about an arthroscopic biceps tenodesis using an interference screw that may not fit through the canula? In these and many other cases, the definitions of "open," "mini-open," and even "arthroscopic" techniques are no longer clear; in many cases, procedures that are normally considered "arthroscopic" are actually "arthroscopically assisted." More confusing is the distinction between mini-open and open approaches based on the size of the incision. As will be discussed in the subsequent chapters, varying degrees of open and arthroscopic techniques exist; there is graying of the borders between them, and several authors have begun publishing instructional monographs on making the transition from one to another, usually toward more minimally invasive techniques [13, 14].

Arthroscopy in Shoulder Surgery

Relatively uniformly in shoulder surgery, the perspective is that the gold standard is open surgery and that arthroscopic or minimally invasive techniques hope to approach these results [15–20]. Ironically, in some cases, minimally invasive surgery may actually have better results than in open cases. This may be due to a distinct advantage of arthroscopy or the lack of a distinct disadvantage inherent in traditional open surgery. Consider the example of rotator cuff repair. Although older reports have shown inferior results with arthroscopic surgery when compared with open surgery, more recent studies have begun to show equivalent results with arthroscopic techniques [15–20]. In the hands of a proficient surgeon, arthroscopy allows for several advantages over open surgery, such as the examination of concomitant intraarticular and subacromial pathology as well as better visualization and releases of both sides of the tendon and the rotator and posterior intervals [13, 14, 21, 22].

Of great concern in any approach to the shoulder is damage to or detachment of the deltoid. In traditional open approaches, the deltoid is elevated off of the acromion and reattached after acromioplasty. Although uncommon, deltoid dehiscence has led to disastrous results, and meticulous repair of the deltoid origin should be done in any open approach. This complication is avoided in mini-open and arthroscopic approaches. As a result, techniques such as the open anterior acromioplasty have relatively fallen by the wayside in favor of arthroscopic subacromial decompression with mini-open rotator cuff repair or even complete arthroscopic approaches [17, 22].

In other cases, concomitant pathology may dictate the surgical approach, as in instability repair. Advantages of arthroscopic repair include preservation of the subscapularis (although splitting the subscapularis in line with its fibers may also accomplish this), ability to thoroughly evaluate and address the entire glenohumeral joint and biceps/superior labrum insertion, less immediate postoperative pain, reduced cost, and improved cosmesis [23, 24]. Disadvantages include difficulty mobilizing large, medialized glenoid bone fragments and repairing capsular tears, especially humeral avulsions [24, 25]. Additionally, minimally invasive approaches may be less helpful in some multidirectional cases where stretching of thin tissue rather than stiffness is more of a concern. Open repair may be necessitated by the need to perform bony procedures and has been advocated for patients with inferior glenoid bone loss who require bone grafting or coracoid transfer, and in patients with very large Hill-Sachs lesions requiring grafting or mini-surface replacement [24, 26–28]. Others continue to recommend open repair for collision athletes, and in revision cases, although this may be debated.

With instability, often revision cases may be performed arthroscopically, especially when failure is due to an unaddressed or improperly (e.g., medial rather than on the glenoid rim) repaired Bankart lesion, while open approaches are used if bone grafting is needed or if subscapularis deficiency requires extensive mobilization and repair or pectoralis major transfer [24, 26–28]. Often in these cases, the procedure may be performed through a concealed axillary, mini-incision approach, as described in the subsequent chapters.

As a result of the blurring of borders between open and minimally invasive approaches, the idea that open surgery is the "gold standard" in the shoulder may not be so black and white any more. Additionally, with excellent results of mini-open and arthroscopic techniques, perhaps the "gold standard" is changing [12, 18, 29]. Regardless of the size or number of incisions

used, the surgeon must be comfortable with whichever approach is chosen and the approach must allow for all necessary pathology to be addressed. As will be seen in the subsequent chapters, excellent results can be achieved with several different techniques, and, for each procedure, there are multiple viable options. Ultimately, each surgeon must decide on an individual and case-by-case basis which approach affords the patient the highest likelihood of the best result with the least chance for complications. In many cases, this will be an all arthroscopic approach. In some cases, best results may still be achieved with traditional open approaches. However, in many cases, the best compromise may come from a minimally invasive open approach, being ever mindful that arthroscopy has not rendered open surgery obsolete. Rather, arthroscopy is yet another tool in the surgeon's armamentarium and it, like any other tool, must be used appropriately in order to ensure the patient the best possible outcome with the least chance for complications.

References

1. Janzing, H. M., Houben, B. J., Brandt, S. E., Chhoeurn, V., Lefever, S., Broos, P., Reynders, P., and Vanderschot, P. The Gotfried Percutaneous Compression Plate versus the Dynamic Hip Screw in the treatment of pertrochanteric hip fractures: minimal invasive treatment reduces operative time and postoperative pain. *J Trauma*, 2002 52(2):293–8
2. Perren, S. M. Evolution of the internal fixation of long bone fractures. The scientific basis of biological internal fixation: choosing a new balance between stability and biology. *J Bone Joint Surg Br*, 2002 84(8):1093–110
3. Schutz, M., Muller, M., Krettek, C., Hontzsch, D., Regazzoni, P., Ganz, R., and Haas, N. Minimally invasive fracture stabilization of distal femoral fractures with the LISS: a prospective multicenter study. Results of a clinical study with special emphasis on difficult cases. *Injury*, 2001 32(Suppl 3): SC48–54
4. Olinger, A., Hildebrandt, U., Mutschler, W., and Menger, M. D. First clinical experience with an endoscopic retroperitoneal approach for anterior fusion of lumbar spine fractures from levels T12 to L5. *Surg Endosc*, 1999 13(12):1215–9
5. Berger, R. A., Deirmengian, C. A., Della Valle, C. J., Paprosky, W. G., Jacobs, J. J., and Rosenberg, A. G. A technique for minimally invasive, quadriceps-sparing total knee arthroplasty. *J Knee Surg*, 2006 19(1):63–70

6. Berger, R. A., Jacobs, J. J., Meneghini, R. M., Della Valle, C., Paprosky, W., and Rosenberg, A. G. Rapid rehabilitation and recovery with minimally invasive total hip arthroplasty. *Clin Orthop Relat Res*, 2004 (429):239–47

7. Goldstein, W. M., Branson, J. J., Berland, K. A., and Gordon, A. C. Minimal-incision total hip arthroplasty. *J Bone Joint Surg Am*, 2003 85-A(Suppl 4):33–8

8. Blaine, T., Voloshin, I., Setter, K., and Bigliani, L. U. Minimally invasive approach to shoulder arthroplasty. In: Scuderi, G. R., Tria, A. J. Jr., and Berger, R. A., (Eds.) *MIS Techniques in Orthopaedics*. New York, NY, Springer, 2006, pp. 45–70

9. Hsu, J., and Galatz, L. M. Mini-incision fixation of proximal humeral four-part fractures. In: Scuderi, G. R., Tria, A. J. Jr., and Berger, R. A., (Eds.) *MIS Techniques in Orthopaedics*. New York, NY, Springer, 2006, pp. 32–44

10. Rhee, Y. G., Ha, J. H., and Cho, N. S. Anterior shoulder stabilization in collision athletes: arthroscopic versus open Bankart repair. *Am J Sports Med*, 2006 34(6):979–85

11. Romeo, A. A., Arciero, R. A., and Conner, P. M. Management of the in-season collision athlete with shoulder instability. In: Burks, R. T. (Ed.) *American Shoulder and Elbow Surgeons/American Orthopaedic Society for Sports Medicine Specialty Day Joint Session*. Proceedings of the 72nd Annual Meeting of the American Academy of Orthopaedic Surgeons, Chicago, IL, 2006

12. Abrams, J. S., and Savoie, F. H. III. Arthroscopic rotator cuff repair: is it the new gold standard? In: *72nd Annual Meeting of the American Academy of Orthopaedic Surgeons*. Washington, DC, 2005, pp. 71

13. Yamaguchi, K., Ball, C. M., and Galatz, L. M. Arthroscopic rotator cuff repair: transition from mini-open to all-arthroscopic. *Clin Orthop Relat Res*, 2001 (390):83–94

14. Yamaguchi, K., Levine, W. N., Marra, G., Galatz, L. M., Klepps, S., and Flatow, E. L. Transitioning to arthroscopic rotator cuff repair: the pros and cons. *Instr Course Lect*, 2003 52:81–92

15. Buess, E., Steuber, K. U., and Waibl, B. Open versus arthroscopic rotator cuff repair: a comparative view of 96 cases. *Arthroscopy*, 2005 21(5):597–604

16. Sauerbrey, A. M., Getz, C. L., Piancastelli, M., Iannotti, J. P., Ramsey, M. L., and Williams, G. R., Jr. Arthroscopic versus mini-open rotator cuff repair: a comparison of clinical outcome. *Arthroscopy*, 2005 21(12):1415–20

17. Severud, E. L., Ruotolo, C., Abbott, D. D., and Nottage, W. M. All-arthroscopic versus mini-open rotator cuff repair: a long-term retrospective outcome comparison. *Arthroscopy*, 2003 19(3):234–8

18. Verma, N. N., Dunn, W., Adler, R. S., Cordasco, F. A., Allen, A., MacGillivray, J., Craig, E., Warren, R. F., and Altchek, D. W. All-arthroscopic versus mini-open rotator cuff repair: a retrospective review with minimum 2-year follow-up. *Arthroscopy*, 2006 22(6):587–94

19. Warner, J. J., Tetreault, P., Lehtinen, J., and Zurakowski, D. Arthroscopic versus mini-open rotator cuff repair: a cohort comparison study. *Arthroscopy*, 2005 21(3):328–32

20. Youm, T., Murray, D. H., Kubiak, E. N., Rokito, A. S., and Zuckerman, J. D. Arthroscopic versus mini-open rotator cuff repair: a comparison of clinical outcomes and patient satisfaction. *J Shoulder Elbow Surg*, 2005 14(5):455–9

21. Baker, C. L., Whaley, A. L., and Baker, M. Arthroscopic rotator cuff tear repair. *J Surg Orthop Adv*, 2003 12(4):175–90

22. Norberg, F. B., Field, L. D., and Savoie, F. H., III. Repair of the rotator cuff. Mini-open and arthroscopic repairs. *Clin Sports Med*, 2000 19(1):77–99

23. Caprise, P. A., Jr. and Sekiya, J. K. Open and arthroscopic treatment of multidirectional instability of the shoulder. *Arthroscopy*, 2006 22(10):1126–31

24. Levine, W. N., Rieger, K., and McCluskey, G. M., III. Arthroscopic treatment of anterior shoulder instability. *Instr Course Lect*, 2005 54:87–96

25. Mohtadi, N. G., Bitar, I. J., Sasyniuk, T. M., Hollinshead, R. M., and Harper, W. P. Arthroscopic versus open repair for traumatic anterior shoulder instability: a meta-analysis. *Arthroscopy*, 2005 21(6):652–8

26. Cole, B. J., Millett, P. J., Romeo, A. A., Burkhart, S. S., Andrews, J. R., Dugas, J. R., and Warner, J. J. Arthroscopic treatment of anterior glenohumeral instability: indications and techniques. *Instr Course Lect*, 2004 53:545–58

27. Millett, P. J., Clavert, P., and Warner, J. J. Open operative treatment for anterior shoulder instability: when and why? *J Bone Joint Surg Am*, 2005 87(2):419–32

28. Salvi, A. E., Paladini, P., Campi, F., and Porcellini, G. The Bristow-Latarjet method in the treatment of shoulder instability that cannot be resolved by arthroscopy. A review of the literature and technical-surgical aspects. *Chir Organi Mov*, 2005 90(4):353–64

29. Bottoni, P. C., Smith, E. L., Berkowitz, M. J., Towle, R. B., and Moore, J. H. Arthroscopic versus open shoulder stabilization for recurrent anterior instability: a prospective randomized clinical trial. *Am J Sports Med*, 2006 34(11):1730–7

Mini-incision Bankart Repair*

Edward W. Lee, Kenneth Accousti,
and Evan L. Flatow

3

Recurrent instability has plagued physicians since ancient times, because this problem can lead to severe disability. The tenuous balance between stability and motion of the glenohumeral joint makes treatment difficult. Historically, surgical procedures to stabilize the shoulder were used mostly for recurrent, locked anterior dislocations. These included staple capsulorraphy [1], subscapularis transposition [2], shortening of the subscapularis and anterior capsule [3], transfer of the coracoid [4], and osteotomies of the proximal humerus [5] or the glenoid neck [6]. Most were successful in the sense of eliminating recurrent dislocations, but often at the cost of restricted external rotation and a resultant risk of late glenohumeral osteoarthrosis [7–11]. Furthermore, the traditional limited operative indications failed to account for the growing awareness of subluxations as a source of symptomatic instability [12–15]. Better understanding of glenohumeral joint biomechanics, the role of the capsuloligamentous structures, and their modes of failure has led to an emphasis on restoration of normal anatomic relationships.

Recent uses of minimally invasive surgery to correct a myriad of orthopedic problems through smaller incisions has included the shoulder, producing a better cosmetic appearance following surgery, and in many cases, providing decreased postoperative pain when compared with similar operations performed through standard incisions.

Anatomy and Biomechanics

The glenohumeral joint has the most range of motion of any articulation in the human body. The lack of bony restraint allows the shoulder to achieve this motion to place the hand in space but this also predisposes the shoulder to instability if the soft tissue capsuloligamentous restraints or osseous architecture is disrupted [16, 17]. The rotator cuff and scapular stabilizers serve as dynamic restraints in normal shoulder biomechanics. A primary role of the rotator cuff is to resist translational forces on the joint through compression of the humeral head into the glenoid cavity.

The glenohumeral joint is composed of a relatively small glenoid that provides little inherent stability. The glenoid labrum helps to deepen the "socket" of the glenohumeral joint and increases stability to the articulation. The three major glenohumeral ligaments function as "check-reins" toward the extremes of motion while remaining relatively lax in the mid-range to allow normal joint translation. Turkel et al. [18] found that the contributions of these structures were position

*Adapted from Lee EW, Flatow EL, Mini-incision Bankart Repair for Shoulder Instability, in Scuderi G, Tria A, Berger R (eds.), *MIS Techniques in Orthopedics*, New York, Springer, 2006, with kind permission of Springer Science and Business Media, Inc.

E.W. Lee (✉)
The CORE Institute, Phoenix, AZ, USA
e-mail: esungyun@gmail.com

dependent. The superior glenohumeral ligament, coracohumeral ligament, and the rotator interval (between the leading edge of the supraspinatus and the superior edge of the subscapularis) restrain anterior humeral head translation in 0° of abduction and external rotation. With increasing abduction to 45°, the middle glenohumeral ligament provides the primary anterior restraint. Finally, the inferior glenohumeral ligament (IGHL) tightens and becomes the prime anterior stabilizer at 90° of abduction and 90° of external rotation. Biomechanical study of the IGHL has demonstrated tensile failure at the glenoid insertion or in midsubstance. Significant deformation, however, was observed in midsubstance even if the ultimate site of failure occurred at the insertion [19].

The anterior–inferior glenoid labrum, with its attachment of the anterior band of the IGHL, provides the primary restraint to anterior humeral translation when the arm is abducted to 90° and externally rotated. The Bankart injury is a disruption of this anterior–inferior labrum and IGHL. In some cases, such as rugby players who dislocate their shoulder while in the "stiff arm" position, traumatic anterior dislocations may result in a fracture of the anterior–inferior glenoid with disruption of the labrum and IGHL. This is termed a bony Bankart injury, and X-ray examination may show a small fragment of bone along the inferior glenoid neck. This fracture can be either an avulsion injury, with the IGHL pulling the inferior glenoid off, or an impaction injury, produced by the humeral head crushing the anterior glenoid lip. This marginal impaction fracture may appear as "missing bone" without a separate fragment anterior and medial to the anterior glenoid rim.

A humeral avulsion of the glenohumeral ligament (HAGL) is a disruption of the glenohumeral ligamentous complex from the humeral neck instead of the more common inferior glenoid. With anterior dislocations, the capsule (with the glenohumeral ligaments) is also stretched and this further increases the laxity of the joint. Commonly, a large pouch of loose capsule filled with synovial fluid will be seen on magnetic resonance imaging (MRI) in patients with instability of the shoulder.

Hill–Sachs lesions can occur after anterior dislocations. This is an impaction fracture on the posterior superior humeral head as the head is compressed on the anterior margin of the glenoid and is akin to a depression (Hill–Sachs) in a ping-pong ball (humeral head). If large enough, these lesions can engage the anterior glenoid rim, leading to instability secondary to loss of congruence of the glenohumeral articulation, in essence, allowing the humeral head to "fall off" the glenoid as the defect engages the anterior rim of the glenoid (engaging Hill–Sachs).

Clinical Features

Patient History

Critical to the evaluation of glenohumeral instability is a careful history and physical examination. The nature of the injury surrounding the onset of symptoms should be determined and are particularly useful in identifying the type of instability. The position of the arm at the time of injury or circumstances that provoke symptoms will often indicate the direction of instability. Reproduction of a patient's symptoms in a position of abduction, external rotation, and extension suggests anterior instability. Flexion, internal rotation, and adduction, in contrast, would more likely point to posterior instability.

In determining the degree and etiology of instability, the history should ascertain whether the initial and any subsequent episodes of instability were elicited by high-energy trauma (such as violent twisting or a fall), minimal repeated trauma (such as throwing a ball), or no trauma (such as reaching for a high shelf). An initial dislocation resulting from a single traumatic episode will frequently produce a Bankart lesion. In contrast, capsular laxity and absence of a Bankart lesion will often be found in those patients who suffer from an atraumatic dislocation, multijoint laxity, and several shoulder subluxations prior to a frank dislocation. The type of reduction required (i.e., was the shoulder self-reduced or did it require manipulation by another person?) may also provide additional information about the extent of joint laxity.

Acquired instability was described by Neer, in which cumulative enlargement of the capsule results from repetitive stress [20]. Overhead-throwing athletes may develop isolated shoulder laxity from overuse with no evidence of laxity in other joints. These patients may become symptomatic after years of microtrauma or only after a frank dislocation following a single traumatic event. This patient group demonstrates that multiple etiologies may contribute to instability and underscores the need for careful diagnosis and treatment to address coexisting pathologic entities.

Voluntary control of instability must be carefully sought out as this may change the ultimate course of treatment. Patients with psychiatric disorders may utilize a concomitant ability to dislocate the shoulder for secondary gain. While operative intervention in this situation would likely fail, treatment options exist for other forms of voluntary subluxation. Surgery may benefit patients who can subluxate the shoulder by placing the arm in provocative positions. Biofeedback techniques, however, may help those patients who sublux through selective muscular activation [21].

A detailed record of prior treatment should also be obtained, including the type and duration of immobilization, rehabilitative efforts, and previous surgeries. Knowledge of failed interventions will help guide future treatment in the recurrent dislocator.

Pain as an isolated symptom will not typically reveal much useful information. Anterior shoulder pain may indicate anterior instability as well as other common disorders including subacromial impingement. Similarly, posterior shoulder pain is nonspecific and may represent a range of pathology from instability to cervical spine disorders. The location of the pain in combination with provoking arm positions and activities, however, may aid in making a diagnosis of instability. Altered glenohumeral kinematics in throwers, for example, may result in posterior shoulder pain during late-cocking ("internal impingement") [22].

Patients may also report other symptoms consistent with subtle shoulder instability. Rowe and Zarins [15] described a phenomenon termed the "dead-arm syndrome" in which paralyzing pain and loss of control of the extremity occurs with abduction and external rotation of the shoulder. A similar phenomenon may be seen in patients with inferior subluxation when they carry heavy loads in the affected arm.

Finally, determining the patient's functional demands and level of impairment is important prior to formulating a therapeutic plan. The different expectations of a sedentary patient with minimal functional loss versus the high-performance athlete with pain and apprehension may affect the type of prescribed treatment.

Physical Examination

A thorough physical examination is equally essential in making an accurate diagnosis and recommending the appropriate intervention. Both shoulders should be adequately exposed and examined for deformity, range of motion, strength, and laxity. Demonstration of scapular winging may accompany instability, particularly of the posterior type, and should be considered a potential cause of symptoms. Generalized ligamentous laxity may also contribute to instability and can be elicited with the ability to touch the thumb to the forearm and hyperextend the index metacarpophalangeal joint beyond 90° (Fig. 3.1). Operative reports and evidence of healed anterior or posterior scars from previous instability repairs will indicate what has been done and may provide a rationale for the patient's current symptoms.

Tenderness to palpation of the acromioclavicular joint should be sought and may represent the source of symptoms in a patient with an asymptomatic loose shoulder. Pain along the glenohumeral joint line can be associated with instability but is a nonspecific finding.

Typically, there is a full range of motion with the exception of guarding at the extremes as the shoulder approaches unstable positions. Clinical suspicion should be raised, however, in the patient older than 40 years of age who is unable to actively abduct the arm after a primary anterior dislocation. It has been shown that a high percentage of these patients will have a concurrent rupture of the rotator cuff with restoration of stability following repair [23].

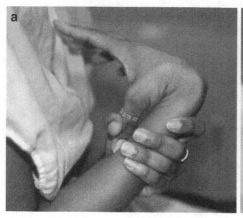
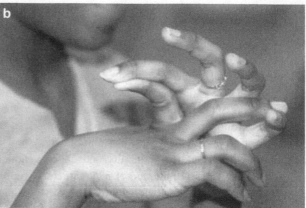

Fig. 3.1 Tests for generalized ligamentous laxity. (**a**) Thumb to forearm. (**b**) Index metacarpophalangeal joint hyperextension (From Lee EW, Flatow EL, Mini-incision Bankart Repair for Shoulder Instability. In: Scuderi G, Tria A, Berger R (eds.), *MIS Techniques in Orthopedics*, New York, Springer, 2006, with kind permission of Springer Science and Business Media, Inc.)

Various basic provocative tests can be used to reproduce the patient's symptoms and confirm the diagnosis. In order to minimize the effects of muscle guarding, these maneuvers should be performed first on the unaffected side and then in succession of increasing discomfort. The *sulcus test* evaluates inferior translation of the humeral head with the arm at the side and in abduction [24] (Fig. 3.2). Significant findings would include an increased palpable gap between the acromion and humeral head compared with the opposite side as well as translation below the glenoid rim. Incompetence of the rotator interval will not reduce the gap with performance of the test in external rotation.

Laxity can be further evaluated by *anterior and posterior drawer* or *load-and-shift tests* [25] (Fig. 3.3). The proximal humerus is shifted in each direction while grasped between the thumb and index fingers. Alternatively, with the patient supine, the scapula is stabilized while the humeral head is axially loaded and translated anteriorly and posteriorly. Translation greater than the opposite shoulder or translation over the glenoid rim indicates significant laxity. Only translations that reproduce the patient's symptoms are considered as demonstrating instability.

The *anterior apprehension test* is performed by externally rotating, abducting, and extending

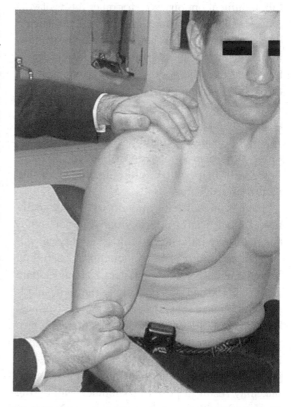

Fig. 3.2 Sulcus sign. Downward traction of the arm will create a gap between the acromion and the humeral head (From Lee EW, Flatow EL, Mini-incision Bankart Repair for Shoulder Instability. In: Scuderi G, Tria A, Berger R (eds.), *MIS Techniques in Orthopedics*, New York, Springer, 2006, with kind permission of Springer Science and Business Media, Inc.)

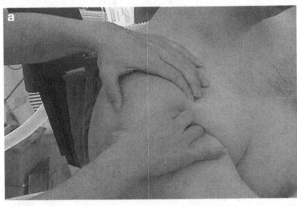
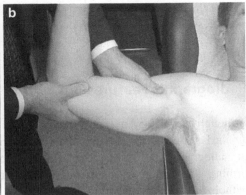

Fig. 3.3 (a) Anterior/posterior drawer: translation of the humeral head between the thumb and index finger and stabilization of the scapula with the other hand. (b) Load and shift: simultaneous axial loading and translation of the humeral head (From Lee EW, Flatow EL, Mini-incision Bankart Repair for Shoulder Instability. In: Scuderi G, Tria A, Berger R (eds.), *MIS Techniques in Orthopedics*, New York, Springer, 2006, with kind permission of Springer Science and Business Media, Inc.)

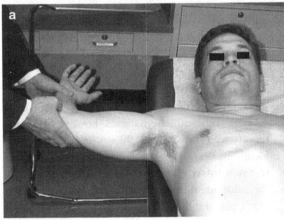
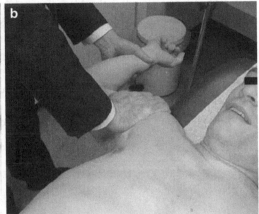

Fig. 3.4 (a) Apprehension test: abduction and external rotation will produce a sense of impending subluxation/dislocation with anterior glenohumeral instability. (b) Relocation test: posterior directed force on the humeral head will alleviate symptoms (From Lee EW, Flatow EL, Mini-incision Bankart Repair for Shoulder Instability. In: Scuderi G, Tria A, Berger R (eds.), *MIS Techniques in Orthopedics*, New York, Springer, 2006, with kind permission of Springer Science and Business Media, Inc.)

the affected shoulder while stabilizing the scapula or providing an anteriorly directed force to the humeral head with the other hand. Significant findings would include a sense of impending subluxation or dislocation, or guarding and resistance to further rotation secondary to apprehension [26] (Fig. 3.4). Pain as an isolated finding is nonspecific and may indicate other pathology such as rotator cuff disease. *Jobe's relocation test* is done in the supine position, usually accompanying the apprehension test. As symptoms are elicited with progressive external rotation, the examiner applies a posteriorly directed force to the humeral head. A positive test is signified by alleviation of symptoms [27] (Fig. 3.4).

Posterior instability can be elicited with the *posterior stress test*. As one hand stabilizes the scapula, a posteriorly directed axial force is applied to the arm with the shoulder in 90° of flexion, and adduction and internal rotation.

Unlike the anterior apprehension test, the posterior stress test will usually produce pain rather than true apprehension [28].

Radiographic Features

Although the history and physical examination are the key elements in patient evaluation, a series of radiographic studies may be helpful in confirming the diagnosis and defining associated pathology. Anteroposterior (AP) radiographs in internal and external rotation, a lateral view in the scapular plane (scapular-Y view), and a lateral of the glenohumeral joint (i.e., a standard supine axillary or Velpeau axillary view) should be obtained in the initial evaluation. A *Hill–Sachs lesion* (posterolateral impression fracture) of the humeral head is best seen on the AP radiograph in internal rotation (Fig. 3.5) or on specialized views such as the Stryker Notch view [29]. Fractures or erosions of the glenoid rim can be detected on an axillary or apical oblique view [30].

Other more specialized imaging studies are not routinely obtained in the initial evaluation of instability but may be useful in a preoperative

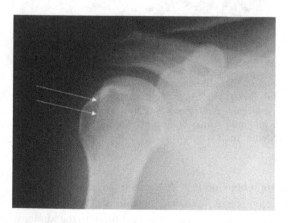

Fig. 3.5 Hill–Sachs lesion. An impaction fracture of the posterolateral humeral head associated with an anterior glenohumeral dislocation is depicted by the *small white arrows* on this internally rotated anteroposterior radiograph (From Lee EW, Flatow EL, Mini-incision Bankart Repair for Shoulder Instability. In: Scuderi G, Tria A, Berger R (eds.), *MIS Techniques in Orthopedics*, New York, Springer, 2006, with kind permission of Springer Science and Business Media, Inc.)

workup. Computed tomography (CT) results can assist in further assessment of fractures and glenoid erosions or altered glenoid version as well as detect subtle subluxation of the humeral head [31, 32]. MRI and magnetic resonance (MR) arthrography can identify associated pathology of the labrum, glenohumeral ligaments, and the rotator cuff [33–35]. The addition of abduction and external rotation has been shown to increase the sensitivity of MR arthrography in delineating tears of the anterior labrum [36, 37]. More recent radiographic modalities such as dynamic MRI currently have no defined indications but may become a useful adjunct in evaluating glenohumeral instability [38].

Nonoperative Treatment

Although the results vary with age and associated bone and soft tissue injury, nonoperative treatment consisting of a period of immobilization followed by rehabilitation is typically successful in managing the majority of patients with glenohumeral instability. Early studies of young (younger than 20 years old), athletic patients, however, found a recurrence rate as high as 90% after a primary dislocation [39, 40]. While subsequent studies have reported lower numbers [41, 42], clearly the risk for subsequent dislocations is higher with earlier onset of instability.

The length and type of immobilization remains a matter of debate. Several published series have advocated immobilization for a few days to several weeks. However, studies by Hovelius [41] and Simonet and Cofield [42] have found no difference in outcome from either the type or length of immobilization. In general, younger patients (younger than 30 years of age) sustaining a primary dislocation are preferably immobilized for approximately 3–4 weeks. Older patients, who have a smaller risk of recurrent instability but a higher susceptibility to stiffness, may be immobilized for shorter periods.

Rehabilitation efforts are aimed at strengthening the dynamic stabilizers and regaining motion. Progressive resistive exercises of the rotator cuff, deltoid, and scapular stabilizers are recommended. Stress on the static restraints (i.e., capsuloligamentous structures) should be prevented in the immediate postinjury period by avoidance of vigorous stretching and provocative arm positions.

Operative Treatment

Failure of conservative management for glenohumeral instability is an indication for proceeding with operative intervention. Open procedures are currently the gold standard for repair of the disrupted soft tissue shoulder stabilizers.

Modern techniques emphasize anatomic restoration of the soft tissue structures. Based on the work of Perthes in 1906 [43], Bankart [44], in 1923, popularized repair of the capsule to the anterior glenoid without shortening of the overlying subscapularis. After modifications to his original description, reconstruction of the avulsed capsule and labrum to the glenoid lip is commonly referred to today as the *Bankart repair*. Several capsulorrhaphy procedures have also been described to address capsular laxity and the increase in joint volume. These procedures allow tightening of the anterior capsule in combination with reattachment of a capsulolabral avulsion.

The inferior capsular shift was first introduced by Neer and Foster for multidirectional instability [24]. This procedure can reduce capsular volume through overlap of capsular tissue on the side of greatest instability and reducing tissue redundancy by tensioning the inferior capsule and opposite side. For anterior inferior instability, we prefer to use a modified inferior capsular shift procedure, in essence a laterally based "T" capsulorrhaphy, which allows us to adapt the repair to each individual [45, 46].

The rationale behind this universal approach to instability is predicated on several factors. First, the capsule is shaped like a funnel with a broader circumferential insertion on the humeral side. Implementing a laterally based incision allows the tissue to be shifted a greater distance and reattached to the broader lateral insertion, thus allowing more capsular overlap. Second, following intraoperative assessment of the inferior pouch and capsular redundancy, the inferior shift procedure permits variable degrees of capsular mobilization around the humeral neck to treat different grades of tissue laxity. Third, use of a "T" capsulorrhaphy permits independent tensioning of the capsule in the medial–lateral and superior–inferior directions. Medial–lateral tensioning is usually a secondary concern, and, if overdone, may result in loss of external rotation. Fourth, a lateral capsular incision affords some protection to the axillary nerve, particularly during an inferior dissection as the nerve traverses under the inferior capsule. Finally, capsular tears/avulsions from the humeral insertion, although rare, are more readily identified and repaired with a laterally based incision.

The patient is placed in a beachchair position, although slightly more recumbent than when performing a rotator cuff repair. We prefer interscalene regional block anesthesia at our institution because of its safety and ability to provide adequate muscle relaxation. Examination under anesthesia should be performed prior to breaching the soft tissues to confirm the predominant components of instability. The key to a "mini-open" Bankart procedure is the use of a concealed anterior axillary incision starting approximately 3 cm below the tip of the coracoid and extending inferiorly for 7–8 cm into the axillary recess (Fig. 3.6). Supplemental local anesthetic is injected into the inferior aspect of the wound where thoracic cross-innervation prevents a complete block in this area. Full-thickness subcutaneous flaps are mobilized until the inferior aspect of the clavicle is palpated. The deltopectoral interval is then developed, taking the cephalic vein laterally with the deltoid. If needed, the upper 1–2 cm of the pectoralis major insertion may be released to gain further exposure. The clavipectoral fascia is then gently incised lateral to the strap muscles, which are gently retracted medially. Osteotomy of the coracoid should not be necessary and may endanger the medial neurovascular structures. A small, medially based wedge of the anterior fascicle of the coracoacromial ligament may be excised to increase visualization of the superior border of the subscapularis muscle, rotator interval, and anterior aspect of the subacromial space.

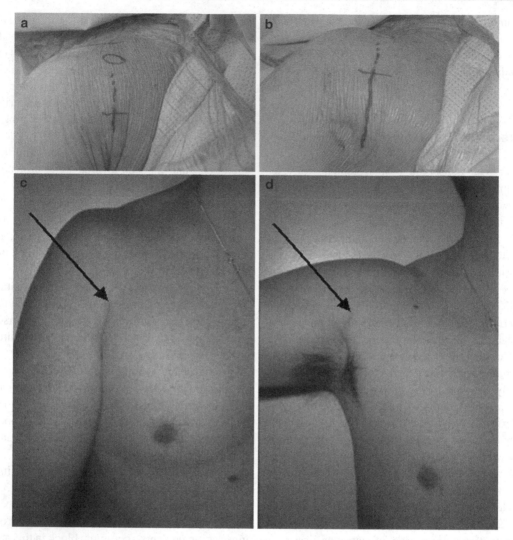

Fig. 3.6 Concealed axillary incision. (**a**) Arm at the side and (**b**) arm in abduction. The *circle* indicates coracoid process. The *solid line* indicates true concealed incision; if needed for more exposure, the *dashed line* indicates extension toward the coracoid. (**c**) and (**d**) Healed axillary incision. *Black arrows* indicate superior extent of incision (From Lee EW, Flatow EL, Mini-incision Bankart Repair for Shoulder Instability. In: Scuderi G, Tria A, Berger R (eds.), *MIS Techniques in Orthopedics*, New York, Springer, 2006, with kind permission of Springer Science and Business Media, Inc.)

The upper and lower borders of the subscapularis are identified. The anterior humeral circumflex vessels are carefully isolated and ligated. Preservation of the inferior border of the subscapularis to provide protection to the axillary nerve has been suggested [47]. This may be a reasonable option in true unidirectional instability cases; however, inadequate exposure of the inferior capsule may compromise the ability to correct any coexisting inferior laxity component.

Another approach splits the subscapularis longitudinally in line with its fibers, making visualization of the glenoid rim more difficult, but motion is less restricted postoperatively. This approach may be useful in athletes who throw, in whom any restriction in external rotation postoperatively should be avoided [48]. We prefer to detach the tendon 1–2 cm from its insertion onto the lesser tuberosity, being careful not to stray too medially into the muscle fibers and compromise the subscapularis repair. Blunt elevation of the muscle belly from the capsule medially may permit easier identification of the plane between the two structures.

Examination of the rotator interval is essential during dissection of the capsule and subscapularis. As one of the primary static stabilizers of the glenohumeral joint, the rotator interval can be an important component of recurrent anterior instability. We repair it when it is widened, aware that overly tightening the gap will limit external rotation.

The capsule is then incised laterally, leaving a 1-cm cuff of tissue for repair while placing traction sutures in the free edge. Placing the arm in adduction and external rotation maximizes the distance between the incision and axillary nerve, which should be palpated and protected throughout the procedure.

The extent of capsular dissection and mobilization will depend on the components of instability. Unidirectional anterior instability will only require dissection of the anterior capsule. Bidirectional anterior–inferior instability will require the addition of inferior capsular mobilization to eliminate the enlarged capsule. In these cases, the shoulder is gradually flexed and externally rotated to facilitate sharp dissection of the anterior and inferior capsule off of the humeral neck. A finger can be placed in the inferior recess to assess the amount of redundant capsule and the adequacy of the shift. As more capsule is mobilized and upward traction is placed on the sutures, the volume of the pouch will reduce and push the finger out, indicating an adequate shift.

The inferior component in unidirectional instability is minimal, and thus, an inferior shift and the horizontal incision may be unnecessary. With a significant inferior capsular redundancy, the horizontal limb of the "T" in the capsule is made between the inferior and middle glenohumeral ligaments. A Fukuda retractor is then placed to visualize the glenoid (Fig. 3.7). If the capsule is thin and redundant medially, a "barrel" stitch can be used to tension it as well as imbricate the capsule at the glenoid rim to serve as an additional bumper to augment a deficient labrum [49] (Fig. 3.8).

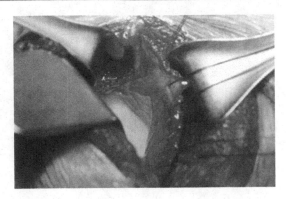

Fig. 3.7 Mobilization of the capsule and placement of traction sutures in the free edge. A Fukuda retractor is placed, allowing inspection of the glenoid (From Lee EW, Flatow EL, Mini-incision Bankart Repair for Shoulder Instability. In: Scuderi G, Tria A, Berger R (eds.), *MIS Techniques in Orthopedics*, New York, Springer, 2006, with kind permission of Springer Science and Business Media, Inc.)

Effectiveness of a shift requires anchoring of the capsule to the glenoid. When the glenohumeral ligaments and labrum are avulsed from the bone medially, they must be reattached to the glenoid rim (Fig. 3.9). The Bankart lesion must be anchored to the rim before performing the capsulorraphy because the capsule must be secured to the glenoid for the shift to be effective. This can be accomplished by inside-out anchoring the labrum with sutures through bone tunnels. After the glenoid rim is roughened with a curette or high-speed burr, two to three sets of holes are made adjacent to the articular surface and through the glenoid rim. Curved awls, angled curettes, and heavy towel clips may be used to fashion the tunnels. A small CurvTek (Arthrotek, Warsaw, IN) may also be helpful in making the holes. Number 0 nonabsorbable braided sutures (e.g., Ethibond [Ethicon/Johnson & Johnson, Somerville, NJ]) are passed through the tunnels. Both limbs are then brought inside-out through the labrum and tied on the outside of the capsule. Alternatively, suture anchors can be utilized, placing them adjacent to the articular margin and careful not to insert them medially to avoid a step–off between the rim and the labrum.

Glenoid deficiency from a fracture of the rim or from repeated wear from chronic instability

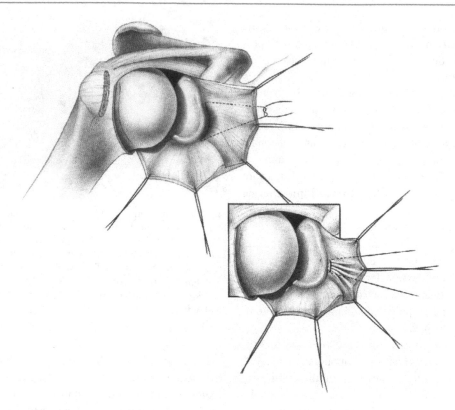

Fig. 3.8 A barrel stitch may be used medially to bunch up tissue at the glenoid rim to compensate for a deficient labrum (From Post M, Bigliani L, Flatow E, et al. The Shoulder: Operative Technique. Philadelphia: Lippincott Williams & Wilkins, 1998, p. 184.)

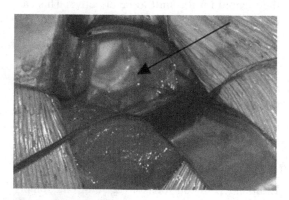

Fig. 3.9 Avulsion of the glenohumeral ligaments and labrum from the glenoid rim. The *solid black arrow* indicates the bare anterior glenoid rim

may contribute to the pathologic process. Defects representing less than 25% of the articular surface area may be repaired by reattaching the labrum and capsule back to the remaining glenoid rim. If a fragment of bone remains attached to the soft tissues, this can be mobilized and repaired back to the glenoid with sutures. Larger fragments can be reattached with a cannulated screw, countersinking the head of the screw within the bone. Defects larger than 25% without a reparable fragment, leaving an "inverted-pear" glenoid in which the normally pear-shaped glenoid had lost enough anterior–inferior bone to assume the shape of an inverted pear [50], should be augmented with bone. Femoral head allograft can be fashioned to reconstitute the rim. Another alternative to deepening the socket is to perform a Bristow–Laterjet procedure, transferring the coracoid tip with the attached coracobrachialis and short head of the biceps into the defect, close to the articular margin and behind the repaired capsule [4]. A cannulated screw, carefully engaging the posterior cortex of the glenoid, and a washer are used to secure the coracoid to the glenoid (Fig. 3.10).

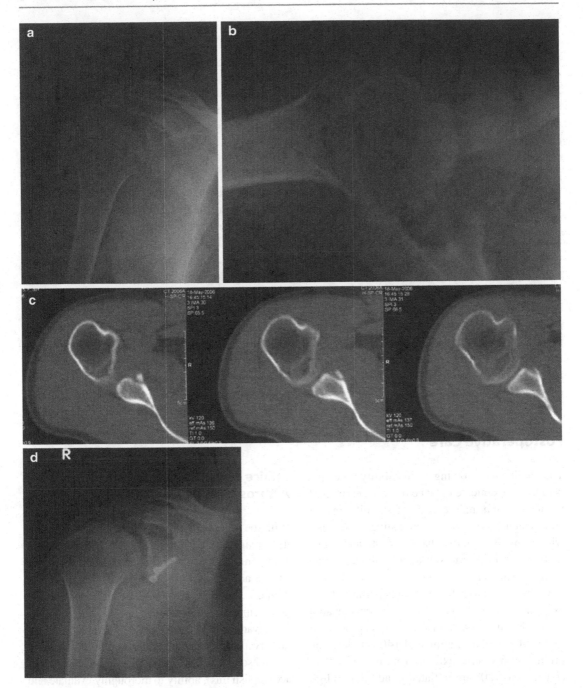

Fig. 3.10 Laterjet coracoid transfer for anterior inferior bony insufficiency. (**a**) and (**b**) Preoperative radiographs. (**c**) Preoperative axial CT images. (**d**) Postoperative scapular anteroposterior and lateral radiograph with bone block and screws in place

An engaging Hill–Sachs lesion may be another source of recurrent instability requiring attention for a successful repair. Preventing the head defect from engaging the glenoid rim can be accom-plished in one of three ways. First, the capsular shift can be performed to tighten the anterior structures enough to restrict external rotation. This should be done with caution as previously mentioned, given the unwanted result in over-head athletes and the risk of late glenohumeral arthrosis. Second, a size-matched humeral osteoarticular allograft or a corticocancellous iliac graft can be utilized to fill the defect. Finally, an internal rotation proximal humeral osteotomy can be performed, albeit with significant technical difficulty and potential morbidity, shifting the defect out of the arc of motion.

To perform the capsular shift, the arm is positioned in at least 20° of external rotation, 30° of abduction, and 10° of flexion while securing the tissues for the capsular shift. In overhead athletes, approximately 10° more abduction and external rotation may be used. Once any adherent soft tissues impeding excursion of the capsule are dissected from the capsule, the inferior flap should be shifted superiorly first, followed by the superior flap to a more inferior position. A suture may be placed medially to reinforce overlap of the two flaps. The subscapularis is then repaired as previously described followed by a layered closure and a subcuticular skin closure.

Postoperative Care

The challenge following an instability procedure is to find the delicate balance between early gradual motion and maintenance of stability. In general, patients are protected in a sling for 6 weeks with immediate active hand, wrist, and elbow motion and isometric shoulder exercises started at approximately 10 days. From 10 days to 2 weeks, gentle assisted motion is permitted with external rotation with a stick to 10° and elevation to 90°. From 2 to 4 weeks, motion is progressed to 30° of external rotation and 140° of elevation. From 4 to 6 weeks, external rotation to 40° and elevation to 160° are initiated in addition to light resistive exercises. Terminal elevation stretching and external rotation to 60° are permitted after 6 weeks. After 3 months, when the soft tissues have adequately healed, terminal external rotation stretches are allowed. Patients can expect a return to sport at 9–12 months postoperatively. These are broad guidelines that should be adapted

to each individual case based on intraoperative findings and frequent postoperative exams. Poor tissue quality, durability of the repair, patient reliability, and future demands on the shoulder should dictate the progression of the rehabilitation program.

Results

Good results have been achieved with most open capsulorraphy techniques to treat anterior/anterior–inferior glenohumeral instability. Thomas and Matsen [51] reported 97% good or excellent results in 63 shoulders with repair of the Bankart lesion and incising both the subscapularis and capsule. Pollock et al. [46] reported 90% successful results with an anterior–inferior capsular shift in 151 shoulders with a 5% rate of recurrent instability. Bigliani et al. [45] studied 68 shoulders in athletes who underwent an anterior–inferior capsular shift with 94% of patients with good or excellent results. Fifty-eight patients (92%) returned to the major sports and 47 patients (75%) returned at the same competitive level.

Choice of Mini-Incision Versus Arthroscopic Repair

With the recent advances in arthroscopic instability repair, failure rates have been comparable to open, mini-incision repair [52, 53]. Many injuries can be addressed by either open or arthroscopic methods, and the limitations of arthroscopic surgery remain controversial.

Advantages of an arthroscopic repair include preservation of the subscapularis (although splitting the subscapularis in line with its fibers may also accomplish this), ability to thoroughly evaluate and visualize the entire glenohumeral joint and biceps/superior labrum insertion, less immediate postoperative pain, reduced cost, and improved cosmesis [54–56]. Disadvantages of an arthroscopic approach include difficulty mobilizing large, medialized glenoid bone fragments and repairing capsular tears, especially humeral avulsions, and the fact that a minimally invasive approach may be less helpful in some multidirectional cases where stretching out of thin tissue rather than stiffness is the most common failure mode. Furthermore, open repair has been advocated for patients with greater than 25% of inferior glenoid bone loss who require bone grafting or coracoid transfer, rare patients with extremely large Hill–Sachs requiring grafting or mini-surface replacement, collision athletes, and revision cases [57–60].

The authors utilize arthroscopic techniques for most cases in which only labral avulsion and capsular stretch needs to be addressed. We will mobilize and repair small glenoid avulsion fragments arthroscopically, but when bone grafting of the glenoid or the Hill–Sachs lesion is required, a mini–incision open approach is employed. Finally, revision cases may be performed arthroscopically in many cases, especially when the failure is due to an unrepaired or improperly (e.g., medial rather than on the glenoid rim) repaired Bankart lesion, but an open approach is used if bone grafting is needed or if subscapularis deficiency from a prior open approach requires extensive mobilization and repair or subcoracoid pectoralis transfer. Usually these procedures may be performed through a concealed axillary, mini-incision approach as previously described.

References

1. Du Toit GT, Roux D. Recurrent dislocation of the shoulder: a twenty-four year study of the Johannesberg stapling operation. *J Bone Joint Surg Am* 38A:1–12, 1956
2. Magnuson PB, Stack JK. Recurrent dislocation of the shoulder. *JAMA* 123:889–92, 1943
3. Clarke HO. Habitual dislocation of the shoulder. *J Bone Joint Surg Br* 30B:19–25, 1948
4. Helfat AJ. Coracoid transplantation for recurring dislocation of the shoulder. *J Bone Joint Surg Br* 40B:198–202, 1958
5. Weber BG, Simpson LA, Hardegger F. Rotational humeral osteotomy for recurrent anterior dislocation of the shoulder associated with a large Hill-Sachs lesion. *J Bone Joint Surg Am* 66(9):1443–50, 1984
6. Saha AK. *Theory of Shoulder Mechanism: Descriptive and Applied.* Springfield, IL, Charles C. Thomas, 1961
7. Hawkins RJ, Angelo RL. Glenohumeral osteoarthrosis. A late complication of the Putti-Platt repair. *J Bone Joint Surg Am* 72(8):1193–7, 1990
8. O'Driscoll SW, Evans DC. Long-term results of staple capsulorrhaphy for anterior instability of the shoulder. *J Bone Joint Surg Am* 75(2):249–58, 1993
9. Samilson RL, Prieto V. Dislocation arthropathy of the shoulder. *J Bone Joint Surg Am* 65(4):456–60, 1983
10. Steinmann SR, Flatow EL, Pollock RG, et al. Evaluation and surgical treatment of failed shoulder instability repairs. In: *38th Annual Meeting of the Orthopaedic Research Society*, p. 727, 1992
11. Young DC, Rockwood CA, Jr. Complications of a failed Bristow procedure and their management. *J Bone Joint Surg Am* 73(7):969–81, 1991
12. Blazina ME, Satzman JS. Recurrent anterior subluxation of the shoulder in athletics: a distinct entity. *J Bone Joint Surg Am* 51A(5):1037–38, 1969
13. Garth WP, Jr, Allman FL, Jr, Armstrong WS. Occult anterior subluxations of the shoulder in noncontact sports. *Am J Sports Med* 15(6):579–85, 1987
14. Hastings DE, Coughlin LP. Recurrent subluxation of the glenohumeral joint. *Am J Sports Med* 9(6):352–5, 1981
15. Rowe CR, Zarins B. Recurrent transient subluxation of the shoulder. *J Bone Joint Surg Am* 63(6):863–72, 1981
16. Levine WN, Flatow EL. The pathophysiology of shoulder instability. *Am J Sports Med* 28(6):910–7, 2000
17. Wang VM, Flatow EL. Pathomechanics of acquired shoulder instability: a basic science perspective. *J Shoulder Elbow Surg* 14(1 Suppl S):2S–11S, 2005
18. Turkel SJ, Panio MW, Marshall JL, Girgis FG. Stabilizing mechanisms preventing anterior dislocation of the glenohumeral joint. *J Bone Joint Surg Am* 63(8):1208–17, 1981
19. Bigliani LU, Pollock RG, Soslowsky LJ, Flatow EL, Pawluk RJ, Mow VC. Tensile properties of the inferior glenohumeral ligament. *J Orthop Res* 10(2):187–97, 1992
20. Neer CS, II. Involuntary inferior and multidirectional instability of the shoulder: etiology, recognition, and treatment. *Instr Course Lect* 34:232–38, 1985
21. Beall MS, Jr, Diefenbach G, Allen A. Electromyographic biofeedback in the treatment of voluntary posterior instability of the shoulder. *Am J Sports Med* 15(2):175–8, 1987
22. Davidson PA, Elattrache NS, Jobe CM, Jobe FW. Rotator cuff and posterior-superior glenoid labrum injury associated with increased glenohumeral motion: a new site of impingement. *J Shoulder Elbow Surg* 4(5):384–90, 1995
23. Neviaser RJ, Neviaser TJ. Recurrent instability of the shoulder after age 40. *J Shoulder Elbow Surg* 4(6):416–8, 1995
24. Neer CS, II, Foster CR. Inferior capsular shift for involuntary inferior and multidirectional instability of the shoulder. A preliminary report. *J Bone Joint Surg Am* 62(6):897–908, 1980
25. Hawkins RJ, Bokor DJ. Clinical evaluation of shoulder problems. In: *The Shoulder*, Rockwood CA, Matsen FA, (eds.), 3rd edition, pp. 149–177. Philadelphia, PA, WB Saunders, 1990

26. Speer KP, Hannafin JA, Altchek DW, Warren RF. An evaluation of the shoulder relocation test. *Am J Sports Med* 22(2):177–83, 1994

27. Jobe FW, Tibone JE, Jobe CM. The shoulder in sports. In: *The Shoulder*, Rockwood CA, Jr, Matsen FA, (eds.), 3rd edition, pp. 961–967. Philadelphia, PA, WB Saunders, 1990

28. Hawkins RJ, Koppert G, Johnston G. Recurrent posterior instability (subluxation) of the shoulder. *J Bone Joint Surg Am* 66(2):169–74, 1984

29. Danzig LA, Greenway G, Resnick D. The Hill-Sachs lesion. An experimental study. *Am J Sports Med* 8(5):328–32, 1980

30. Garth WP, Jr, Slappey CE, Ochs CW. Roentgenographic demonstration of instability of the shoulder: the apical oblique projection. A technical note. *J Bone Joint Surg Am* 66(9):1450–3, 1984

31. Itoi E, Lee SB, Amrami KK, Wenger DE, An KN. Quantitative assessment of classic anteroinferior bony Bankart lesions by radiography and computed tomography. *Am J Sports Med* 31(1):112–8, 2003

32. Nyffeler RW, Jost B, Pfirrmann CW, Gerber C. Measurement of glenoid version: conventional radiographs versus computed tomography scans. *J Shoulder Elbow Surg* 12(5):493–6, 2003

33. Beltran J, Rosenberg ZS, Chandnani VP, Cuomo F, Beltran S, Rokito A. Glenohumeral instability: evaluation with MR arthrography. *Radiographics* 17(3):657–73, 1997

34. Parmar H, Jhankaria B, Maheshwari M, Singrakhia M, Shanbag S, Chawla A, Deshpande S. Magnetic resonance arthrography in recurrent anterior shoulder instability as compared to arthroscopy: a prospective comparative study. *J Postgrad Med* 48(4):270–3; discussion 273–4, 2002

35. Shankman S, Bencardino J, Beltran J. Glenohumeral instability: evaluation using MR arthrography of the shoulder. *Skeletal Radiol* 28(7):365–82, 1999

36. Cvitanic O, Tirman PF, Feller JF, Bost FW, Minter J, Carroll KW. Using abduction and external rotation of the shoulder to increase the sensitivity of MR arthrography in revealing tears of the anterior glenoid labrum. *AJR Am J Roentgenol* 169(3):837–44, 1997

37. Wintzell G, Larsson H, Larsson S. Indirect MR arthrography of anterior shoulder instability in the ABER and the apprehension test positions: a prospective comparative study of two different shoulder positions during MRI using intravenous gadodiamide contrast for enhancement of the joint fluid. *Skeletal Radiol* 27(9):488–94, 1998

38. Allmann KH, Uhl M, Gufler H, Biebow N, Hauer MP, Kotter E, Reichelt A, Langer M. Cine-MR imaging of the shoulder. *Acta Radiol* 38(6):1043–6, 1997

39. Rowe CR. Prognosis in dislocations of the shoulder. *J Bone Joint Surg Am* 38A:957–77, 1956

40. Wheeler JH, Ryan JB, Arciero RA, Molinari RN. Arthroscopic versus nonoperative treatment of acute shoulder dislocations in young athletes. *Arthroscopy* 5(3):213–7, 1989

41. Hovelius L. Anterior dislocation of the shoulder in teenagers and young adults. Five-year prognosis. *J Bone Joint Surg Am* 69(3):393–9, 1987

42. Simonet WT, Cofield RH. Prognosis in anterior shoulder dislocation. *Am J Sports Med* 12(1):19–24, 1984

43. Perthes G. Uber operationen bei habitueller schulterluxation. *Deutsch Ztschr Chir* 85:199–227, 1906

44. Bankart ASB. Recurrent or habitual dislocation of the shoulder joint. *Br Med J* 2:1132–35, 1923

45. Bigliani LU, Kurzweil PR, Schwartzbach CC, Wolfe IN, Flatow EL. Inferior capsular shift procedure for anterior-inferior shoulder instability in athletes. *Am J Sports Med* 22(5):578–84, 1994

46. Pollock RG, Owens JM, Nicholson GP, et al. Anterior inferior capsular shift procedure for anterior glenohumeral instability: long term results. In: *39th Annual Meeting of the Orthopaedic Research Society*, p. 974, 1993

47. Matsen FA, III, Thomas SC, Rockwood CA, Jr, Wirth MA. Glenohumeral instability. In: *The Shoulder*, Rockwood CA, Jr, Matsen FA, (eds.), 3rd edition, pp. 611–754. Philadelphia, PA, WB Saunders, 1998

48. Rubenstein DL, Jobe FW, Glousman RE, et al. Anterior capsulolabral reconstruction of the shoulder in athletes. *J Shoulder Elbow Surg* 1:229–37, 1993

49. Ahmad CS, Freehill MQ, Blaine TA, Levine WN, Bigliani LU. Anteromedial capsular redundancy and labral deficiency in shoulder instability. *Am J Sports Med* 31(2):247–52, 2003

50. Burkhart SS, De Beer JF. Traumatic glenohumeral bone defects and their relationship to failure of arthroscopic Bankart repairs: significance of the inverted-pear glenoid and the humeral engaging Hill-Sachs lesion. *Arthroscopy* 16(7):677–94, 2000

51. Thomas SC, Matsen FA, III. An approach to the repair of avulsion of the glenohumeral ligaments in the management of traumatic anterior glenohumeral instability. *J Bone Joint Surg Am* 71(4):506–13, 1989

52. Carreira DS, Mazzocca AD, Oryhon J, Brown FM, Hayden JK, Romeo AA. A prospective outcome evaluation of arthroscopic Bankart repairs: minimum 2-year follow-up. *Am J Sports Med* 34(5):771–7, 2006

53. Tjoumakaris FP, Abboud JA, Hasan SA, Ramsey ML, Williams GR. Arthroscopic and open Bankart repairs provide similar outcomes. *Clin Orthop Relat Res* 446:227–32, 2006

54. Abrams JS, Savoie FH, III, Tauro JC, Bradley JP. Recent advances in the evaluation and treatment of shoulder instability: anterior, posterior, and multidirectional. *Arthroscopy* 18(9 Suppl 2):1–13, 2002

55. Sachs RA, Williams B, Stone ML, Paxton L, Kuney M. Open Bankart repair: correlation of results with postoperative subscapularis function. *Am J Sports Med* 33(10):1458–62, 2005

56. Wang C, Ghalambor N, Zarins B, Warner JJ. Arthroscopic versus open Bankart repair: analysis of patient subjective outcome and cost. *Arthroscopy* 21(10):1219–22, 2005

57. Boileau P, Villalba M, Hery JY, Balg F, Ahrens P, Neyton L. Risk factors for recurrence of shoulder instability after arthroscopic Bankart repair. *J Bone Joint Surg Am* 88(8):1755–63, 2006
58. Mazzocca AD, Brown FM, Jr, Carreira DS, Hayden J, Romeo AA. Arthroscopic anterior shoulder stabilization of collision and contact athletes. *Am J Sports Med* 33(1):52–60, 2005
59. Pagnani MJ, Dome DC. Surgical treatment of traumatic anterior shoulder instability in American football players. *J Bone Joint Surg Am* 84A(5):711–5, 2002
60. Rhee YG, Ha JH, Cho NS. Anterior shoulder stabilization in collision athletes: arthroscopic versus open Bankart repair. *Am J Sports Med* 34(6):979–85, 2006

Mini-open Rotator Cuff Repair

W. Anthony Frisella and Frances Cuomo

Rotator cuff pathology is a common cause of shoulder pain and disability, and becomes more common with advancing patient age. Most symptomatic rotator cuff disease is seen in patients in their fifth and sixth decades. Tears of the rotator cuff are associated with pain and weakness and can result in significant disability [1]. However, it is also known that asymptomatic rotator cuff tears exist in a large percentage of patients, and the presence of asymptomatic tears increases with increasing age [1, 2]. The cause of a tear of the rotator cuff is debated, but is most likely related to a combination of several factors: (1) impingement against the subacromial arch, (2) age-related degeneration or atrophy, (3) overuse, and (4) trauma [1, 3]. The rationale for repairing the torn rotator cuff is derived from multiple published studies demonstrating improved function and decreased pain after rotator cuff repair and rehabilitation. Although complete healing of the tendon does not always occur, rotator cuff repair is recognized as a beneficial procedure by (1) relieving pain, (2) improving strength, and (3) improving range of motion in the affected shoulder. The earliest report of rotator cuff repair comes from Codman in 1911 [4]. Since then, many studies have demonstrated good outcomes with improved pain and function following formal open repair of the rotator cuff with decompression of the subacromial space and acromioplasty [5–12]. The method by which the cuff is repaired, however, has changed over the past two decades, with a movement toward minimally invasive techniques, including both mini-open and arthroscopic repair. The mini-open or deltoid-splitting approach to the rotator cuff is a well-characterized procedure with excellent outcomes and is a useful and successful method of rotator cuff repair.

Arthroscopic visualization of joints was first described in 1931, and the advent of shoulder arthroscopy in the 1980s fundamentally changed the approach to diagnosis and treatment of pathology, including rotator cuff tears [13–15]. The rotator cuff could be visualized arthroscopically and tears could be identified and characterized. The ability to visualize the anatomy of the shoulder through the arthroscope inevitably led to strategies to treat rotator cuff tears by less invasive means. Prior to arthroscopy, rotator cuff tears were treated by formal open repair with approaches that violated the deltoid insertion on the acromion. The deltoid was removed from the acromion in order to perform an acromioplasty and decompression, and repaired to the acromion at the end of the procedure. This approach carried the risk of deltoid avulsion, a rare but catastrophic complication [16–18]. Diagnosis and characterization of tears by arthroscopy led to the description of the arthroscopically assisted, mini-open, or deltoid-splitting repair technique of rotator cuff repair [19]. The success of the mini-open technique was followed by the description of

W.A. Frisella (✉)
Department of Orthopedics and Sports Medicine,
Beth Israel Medical Center, Philips Ambulatory
Care Center, New York, NY, USA
e-mail: anthonyfrisella@gmail.com

G.R. Scuderi and A.J. Tria (eds.), *Minimally Invasive Surgery in Orthopedics: Upper Extremity Handbook*,
DOI 10.1007/978-1-4614-0673-0_4, © Springer Science+Business Media, LLC 2012

completely arthroscopic rotator cuff repair, which has also been successful. However, mini-open repair remains a viable alternative to arthroscopic repair and has advantages over both arthroscopic and formal open repair.

The mini-open rotator cuff repair represents a bridge between open and arthroscopic rotator cuff repair. It has specific advantages and disadvantages when compared with other methods of cuff repair. Advantages over open repair include the adjunctive use of arthroscopy for diagnosis and characterization of the torn cuff tendon as well as identification and treatment of associated shoulder pathology [20, 21]. The arthroscopic portion of the procedure can also be used to mark the torn tendon and to assist in performing the repair. In addition, the deltoid origin is minimally disturbed, allowing for faster rehabilitation and greatly decreasing the possibility of deltoid avulsion as a complication. Mini-open repair creates less surgical trauma, facilitating early hospital discharge and decreasing postoperative pain.

Mini-open repair also has advantages over arthroscopic repair. The primary advantage is the avoidance of complex arthroscopic suture passing and tying techniques. An additional advantage of the mini-open repair is its usefulness as a bridge between the formal open and completely arthroscopic repair techniques, allowing the surgeon a means of gradual transition between the two, if desired. Like arthroscopic repair, mini-open repair with adjunctive arthroscopy allows for direct visualization of the glenohumeral joint and subacromial space for the purposes of diagnosis and allows for the performance of adjunctive arthroscopic procedures, e.g., subacromial decompression, arthroscopic releases, and glenohumeral debridement. Direct arthroscopic visualization of the cuff allows the surgeon to characterize the size and orientation of the tear prior to repair. In addition, mini-open repairs have similar morbidity rates when compared with arthroscopic repairs.

Technique

There are many variations of the technique of mini-open rotator cuff repair. The basic principles are the same, however, and the steps are as follows. First, the shoulder is examined under anesthesia. The patient is then positioned and the shoulder prepped and draped as for arthroscopy. A complete diagnostic arthroscopy is performed and the presence of a cuff tear is confirmed. Associated intraarticular pathology is addressed as necessary. The subacromial space is then entered and a subacromial decompression and acromioplasty are performed. The lateral arthroscopy portal incision is then extended and the deltoid is split, exposing the cuff tear. Open repair of the tear is then performed. These steps are a general guideline. The specific approach to mini-open repair used in our center is described in detail in this section.

The patient is placed supine on the operating table. Regional anesthesia is administered, typically an interscalene block (Fig. 4.1), and may be the only anesthesia given. A light general anesthesia may be used in addition for patient comfort or per patient preference. Once adequate anesthesia is obtained, an examination under anesthesia is performed to document full range of motion. Secondary stiffness may develop in patients with rotator cuff tears, making it important to document adequate range of motion prior to the start of the procedure. If the patient has a stiff shoulder, a manipulation may be performed to release adhesions. The patient is then ready for positioning in the beachchair or sitting position. The beach chair position is characterized by (1) elevation of the torso so that the acromion is parallel to the floor, (2) elevation of the thighs above the buttocks, and (3) flexion of the knees to a comfortable position. In this position, the buttocks are in the most dependent position, ensuring that the patient is stable and will not slip down the table. The surgeon must have adequate access to the posterior shoulder to the medial border of the scapula and the anterior shoulder to the level of the mid-clavicle. The head is held gently in place with a head holder. Generally, specialized table attachments are available to facilitate adequate exposure by dropping the back of the table away from the operative shoulder.

The shoulder is prepped and draped with care taken to ensure exposure of the widest area possible, especially posteriorly. "Draping yourself out" is a common and frustrating occurrence for

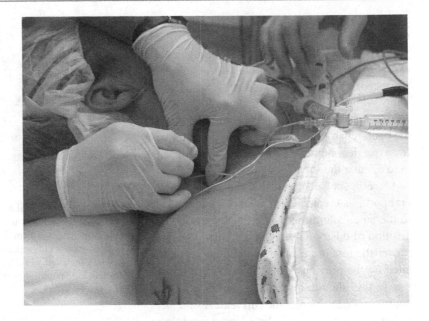

Fig. 4.1 Interscalene block is placed prior to examination under anesthesia. A general anesthesia can be used in place of, or in addition to, regional anesthesia

the inexperienced shoulder arthroscopist. A standard posterior portal is created. Finding the correct position of this portal in the medial-lateral direction may be facilitated by feeling the notch in the spine of the scapula. The slight indentation that can be palpated along the posterior spine is usually about 2 cm medial to the posterolateral corner of the acromion. The portal is then placed about 2 cm inferior to this point. A blunt trocar is used to penetrate the posterior capsule and a diagnostic arthroscopy is begun.

If necessary, an anterior portal can be created. Creation of this portal is facilitated by placing a spinal needle into the rotator interval beneath the course of the biceps tendon, above the subscapularis muscle. A thorough diagnostic arthroscopy is then performed. The glenohumeral articulation is examined for lesions and cartilage loss. The superior labrum is inspected and palpated along with the biceps tendon anchor. The anterior and inferior labrum are inspected with their associated middle and inferior glenohumeral ligaments. The axillary recess is examined, followed by the posterior labrum. Pathology is addressed as necessary, but is beyond the scope of this chapter.

Once an adequate diagnostic arthroscopy of the rest of the joint is undertaken, attention is turned to the rotator cuff. The cuff insertion is examined, starting with the anterior border of the

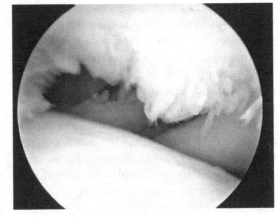

Fig. 4.2 The torn edge of the rotator cuff can be seen from the glenohumeral joint. The humeral head is inferior and the biceps tendon can be seen to the right. Most tears begin just posterior to the biceps tendon

supraspinatus tendon adjacent to the exit of the biceps tendon from the joint (Fig. 4.2). The anterior border of the supraspinatus is the starting point for most degenerative tears and must always be carefully examined. Partial-thickness tears may also be identified here, characterized by pulling away of the articular side of the cuff from its insertion. Once the cuff tear is identified, the edges of the cuff should be debrided. Gentle debridement with a shaver may facilitate an inflammatory response that enhances healing. Debridement may also be used simply to facilitate visualization of the tear. The defect in the cuff may be marked with a percutaneously placed spinal needle, especially for a partial-thickness tear. A suture is advanced through the needle into the glenohumeral joint, allowing easier identification during the subacromial portion of the procedure and during the open repair. The arthroscope is then removed from the glenohumeral joint and the blunt trocar is used to enter the subacromial space.

Once in the subacromial space, an anterolateral portal is created 2 cm posterior and inferior to the anterolateral border of the acromion. The position of this portal may be modified to center it over the rotator cuff tear, which may be facilitated by the previously placed marking suture – the suture should be exiting the skin at the approximate location of the cuff tear. A skin incision is made in Langer's lines and a cannula is introduced and visualized in the subacromial space. There has been some controversy about the necessity of performing a subacromial decompression in the context of a rotator cuff tear. Nevertheless, we routinely perform a subacromial decompression, release the coracoacromial (CA) ligament, and perform an acromioplasty prior to cuff repair. The tear is identified using the previously placed marking suture, and further debridement is undertaken in the lateral gutter of the subacromial space. A thorough bursectomy, especially laterally, will facilitate visualization of the tear during the open portion of the procedure. The tendon edges may again be lightly debrided with a shaver.

At this point, traction sutures may be placed arthroscopically through the edge of the cuff. This may be a useful step for the surgeon who is transitioning from open to arthroscopic repairs. The arthroscopically placed sutures may then be used as traction sutures during the open portion of the repair. Alternatively, the arthroscopic portion of the procedure can be terminated and attention turned to exposure of the rotator cuff. Arthroscopic instruments are removed and the anterolateral skin incision is extended horizontally at both ends to a total distance of 3–4 cm. The incision should be extended in such a way as to make exposure of the tear easier and thus minimize the length of

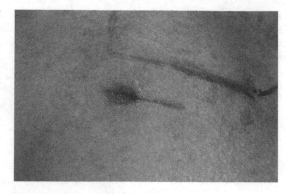

Fig. 4.3 The lateral portal is extended horizontally in line with Langer's lines. The total distance of the incision is usually between 3 and 4 cm (From Schneider JA, Cuomo F, Mini-open rotator cuff repair. In: Scuderi GR, Tria AJ, Jr., (eds.), *MIS Techniques in Orthopedics*, New York, Springer, 2006, with kind permission of Springer Science + Business Media, Inc.)

skin incision (Fig. 4.3). The skin is undermined and freed from the underlying deltoid fascia. The deltoid is then split in line with its fibers, incorporating the previous arthroscopic puncture into the split. The split in the deltoid has two limits. First, the deltoid insertion should be protected and dissection should not lift the deltoid off the acromion. Second, the split in the deltoid should not extend further distal than 4 cm from the edge of the acromion to avoid injury to the axillary nerve. The nerve is located, on average, 6.3 cm from the edge of the acromion on the deep surface of the deltoid [22], but occasionally can be found much closer.

Once the deltoid is split, the subacromial space is entered. Blunt self-retaining retractors may be helpful to hold the fibers of the deltoid apart, but care should be taken to avoid excess pressure and deltoid necrosis. Further bursectomy may be necessary to visualize the tear. Appropriate rotation of the arm is the key to positioning the cuff tear underneath the deltoid split. By varying the position of the arm, different portions of the cuff can be brought into view. If the tear is large and traction sutures had not already been placed, they can be placed to help mobilize the cuff and allow easier repair. Multiple large traction sutures can be placed through the cuff using simple stitches (Fig. 4.4). Traction sutures allow the cuff to be

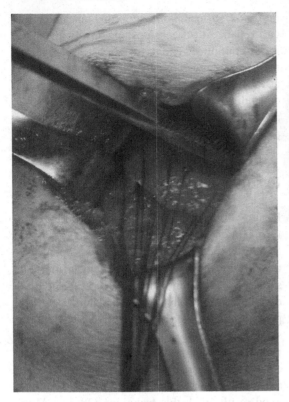

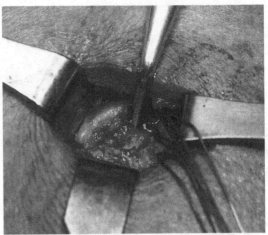

Fig. 4.5 Preparation of the greater tuberosity has been accomplished by debriding away soft tissue. Here an awl is used to create a tunnel for transosseous suture placement

Fig. 4.4 Traction sutures have been placed into the tendon to mobilize it. Traction on the tendon allows for easier releases and better tendon excursion. The goal is to repair the tendon to bone with no tension while the arm is at the side

manipulated for releases, further suture placement, and to relieve tension while tying the definitive suture.

Extraarticular adhesions are released, allowing the cuff to be fully mobilized. The goal of release is to gain enough mobility to allow a tension-free repair with the arm at the side. Intraarticular adhesions deep to the cuff as well as the coracohumeral ligament may need to be addressed, and they can be transected as necessary. Once adequate mobilization is obtained, the size and shape of the tear is again evaluated. U-shaped tears can be repaired with a combination of side-to-side sutures and bone fixation while crescent-shaped tears are generally repaired directly to bone. Once side-to-side sutures are placed, a smaller cuff edge will be left for attachment to bone. Attention is then turned to the greater tuberosity (Fig. 4.5). The tuberosity is cleared of soft tissue, but decortication is not necessary.

This is supported by the work of St. Pierre [23], which showed in a goat model that tendon could be repaired to either cortical or cancellous bone with equal strength and equivalent histological evidence of healing.

Bony fixation can be accomplished either through transosseous tunnels or suture anchors. Bone tunnels or suture anchors are placed in the anatomic insertion or "footprint" of the cuff, and their position is chosen to allow an even repair of the tendon edge without bunching or excessive tension on one portion of the cuff. If using suture anchors, double-row fixation may be considered to better reapproximate the anatomic insertion of the cuff and to provide a stronger repair [24, 25]. For cuff stitches, a grasping stitch such as a modified Mason-Allen has higher pullout strength when compared with simple or horizontal mattress sutures [26]. Generally, braided #2 nonabsorbable sutures are used for repair. Once the anchors or drill holes have been placed and the cuff sutured, the free suture ends are sequentially tied (Fig. 4.6). The previously placed traction sutures can be used to hold the cuff in place, without tension, and removed after tying is complete. Once the cuff has been repaired, the shoulder is taken through a range of motion to demonstrate the safe range for rehabilitation.

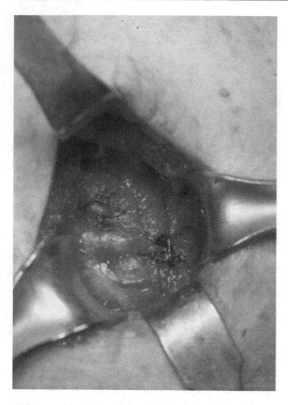

Fig. 4.6 The cuff is repaired with transosseous sutures securely down to bone

The wound is thoroughly irrigated and the deltoid fascia is meticulously repaired. A subcutaneous and subcuticular closure is performed and dressings are applied.

Postoperative Protocol

The patient is discharged from the hospital on the day of surgery. The patient is placed in a sling and is allowed out of the sling only for physical therapy exercises. Passive range-of-motion exercises are begun within the safe range documented at the time of surgery, including forward elevation, external rotation, and pendulum exercises. Internal rotation is not allowed until the cuff has healed. Elbow and hand exercises are also begun. The patient performs pendulum, elbow, and wrist exercises at home several times a day, while passive motion exercises are performed either at home or formally with physical therapy several times a week. The goal of early rehabilitation is to minimize stiffness without putting tension on the cuff repair. At 6 weeks postoperatively, the sling is discontinued and active-assisted range-of-motion exercises are added. Strengthening exercises are begun at 8–12 weeks postoperatively, depending on the size of the tear. A strengthening and stretching program is continued until 1 year postoperatively.

Results

Historically, good results have been reported after formal open repair of rotator cuff tears [5–8, 12]. Similarly, the reported results of mini-open rotator cuff repairs have been excellent in multiple series. An early report from Levy et al. in 1990 demonstrated excellent or good results in 80% of patients and a satisfaction rate of 96% [19]. In the same year, Paulos et al. reviewed a series of 18 patients and reported 88% good or excellent outcomes and minimal complications [27]. Later reports from multiple authors revealed similar good results with this technique [28–31]. More recently, Park et al. reported on a series of 110 small or medium-sized rotator cuff repairs performed with an arthroscopically assisted mini-open technique. Excellent or satisfactory results were reported in 96% of patients at 3-year follow-up. They attributed the majority of their poor results (of which there were only four) to failure to address acromioclavicular joint pathology at the time of cuff repair [32]. Hersch et al. published a series of 22 mini-open repairs in patients with moderate- to large-sized tears. These patients were followed an average of 40 months and demonstrated improvement in the Constant, UCLA, and ASES scores, with a high satisfaction rate of 86% [33]. The report by Shinners et al. in 2002 also demonstrated good results in a larger cohort of 41 patients at 3-year follow-up [34].

Longer follow-up has confirmed the durability of this procedure. Posada et al. examined a cohort of patients at both 2 and 5 years after mini-open repair. Equivalent clinical outcome scores were reported at both follow-ups, demonstrating that the benefit of the procedure does not deteriorate with time [35]. A similar study examining patients at 2- and 7-year follow-up demonstrated good-to-excellent results in 74% of patients at 2 years and 84% at 7 years. Again, good results were maintained or improved with time [36].

Several studies have compared formal open with mini-open repairs. In general, results have been comparable between the two procedures. In 1995, Baker reported on 37 shoulders, comparing 20 open repairs with 17 done through a mini-open incision. The two groups were comparable in terms of size of tear, and postoperative patient satisfaction was the same. Patients with repairs done through a mini-open approach spent less time in the hospital and they returned to work earlier [37]. Other studies have shown similar results between open and mini-open repairs [38–40]. The study by Hata et al. in 2001 showed an earlier return to activities and earlier restoration of range of motion following mini-open repair when compared with formal open repair [39]. To summarize, the published experience of mini-open rotator cuff repair demonstrates a high proportion of good to excellent results, with minimal complications in multiple small to medium series. In addition, results are comparable to open repair with earlier return of function and shorter hospital stays.

Multiple recent studies have compared the results of mini-open repair with all-arthroscopic repair of rotator cuff tears [40–44]. Ide et al. compared two groups of 50 patients who underwent either mini-open or all-arthroscopic repair. The two groups were similar in terms of the size of the cuff tear, and the outcomes as measured by the UCLA score were equivalent. Verma et al. and Youm et al. both published similar series showing the same result: equivalence of mini-open and all-arthroscopic rotator cuff repairs [43, 44]. Finally, Buess et al. compared a group of patients who had mini-open and formal open repair with a second group of patients who had arthroscopic repair. The groups had similar outcomes, but the results of this study are difficult to extrapolate to mini-open repairs as both mini-open and formal open repairs were combined into one group [41]. All of these studies demonstrate methodological problems and to date no randomized controlled trial has compared outcomes for these two surgical procedures. A large multicenter randomized controlled trial is currently underway in Canada to compare mini-open with arthroscopic rotator cuff repair in small to moderate-sized tears [45]. Based on their power analysis, a total of 250 patients will be enrolled in order to detect a clinically significant difference between the two groups. This trial represents the first attempt to definitely compare the results of these two procedures.

Summary

Mini-open rotator cuff repair is a very successful procedure with multiple published studies demonstrating a high proportion of good-to-excellent results using well-validated outcomes measures. The technique is less technically demanding than all-arthroscopic repair while still retaining the advantages of arthroscopic repair. These include the ability to perform diagnostic arthroscopy, preservation of the deltoid origin, faster hospital discharge, less postoperative pain, and subsequent accelerated rehabilitation. Mini-open repair seems to be approximately equivalent to all-arthroscopic repair in multiple nonrandomized comparative studies, and a randomized trial is underway to formally address this question. Mini-open repair remains a viable option for the surgeon who wishes to use classic surgical suture passing and tying while also taking advantage of arthroscopic examination and treatment of the shoulder joint. Although there is a current trend toward using arthroscopic repair, there is no published evidence that definitively demonstrates its superiority over the mini-open procedure. The mini-open approach should remain a useful tool for rotator cuff repair for the foreseeable future.

References

1. Matsen FA, Arntz CT. Rotator cuff tendon failure. In: Rockwood CA, Matsen FA, eds. *The Shoulder.* Philadelphia: Harcourt Brace Jovanovich, Inc. 1990:647–665
2. Yamaguchi K, Middleton WD, Hildebolt CF et al. The demographic and morphological features of rotator cuff disease. A comparison of asymptomatic and symptomatic shoulders. J Bone Joint Surg 2006;88: 1699–1704

3. Neer CS II. Anterior acromioplasty for the chronic impingement syndrome in the shoulder: a preliminary report. J Bone Joint Surg Am 1972;53:41–50

4. Codman EA. Complete rupture of the supraspinatous tendon: operative treatment with report of two successful cases. Boston Med Surg J 1911;164:708–710

5. Packer NP, Calvert PT, Bayley JIL et al. Operative treatment of chronic ruptures of the rotator cuff of the shoulder. J Bone Joint Surg Br 1983;65(B):171–175

6. Hawkins RJ, Misamore GW, Hobelka PE. Surgery for full thickness rotator cuff tears. J Bone Joint Surg Am 1985;67:1349–1355

7. Neer CS II, Flatow EL, Lech O. Tears of the rotator cuff. Long term results of anterior acromioplasty and repair. Orthop Trans 1988;12:735

8. Ellman H, Hanker G, Bayer M. Repair of the rotator cuff. End-result study of factors influencing reconstruction. J Bone Joint Surg Am 1986;68:1136–1144

9. Ellman H, Kay SP. Arthroscopic subacromial decompression for chronic impingement. Two to five year results. J Bone Joint Surg Br 1991;73:395–398

10. Gazielly DF, Gleyze P, Montagnon C. Functional and anatomical results of rotator cuff repair. Clin Orthop Relat Res 1994;304:43–53

11. Gupta R, Leggin BG, Iannotti JP. Results of surgical repair of full thickness tears of the rotator cuff. Orthop Clin North Am 1997;28:241–248

12. Bigliani L, Cordasco F, McIlveen S et al. Operative treatment of massive rotator cuff tears: long-term results. J Shoulder Elbow Surg 1992;1:120–130

13. Burman MS. Arthroscopy or the direct visualization of joints: an experimental cadaver study. J Bone Joint Surg Am 1931;13:669–695

14. Wantanabe M. Arthroscopy of the shoulder joint. In: Wantanabe M, ed. Arthroscopy of Small Joints. Tokyo: Igaku-Shoin;1985:45–46

15. Wiley AM, Older MB. Shoulder arthroscopy: investigations with a fibro-optic instrument. Am J Sports Med 1980;8:18

16. Yamaguchi K. Complications of rotator cuff repair. Tech Orthop 1997;12:33–41

17. Mansat P, Cofield RH, Kersten TE et al. Complications of rotator cuff repair. Orthop Clin North Am 1997;28:205–213

18. Karas EH, Iannotti JP. Failed repair of the rotator cuff: evaluation and treatment of complications. Instr Course Lect 1998;47:87–95

19. Levy HJ, Uribe JW, Delaney LG. Arthroscopic assisted rotator cuff repair: preliminary results. Arthroscopy 1990;6:55–60

20. Gartsman GM, Taverna E. The incidence of glenohumeral joint abnormalities associated with full thickness, repairable rotator cuff tears. Arthroscopy 1997;13:450–455

21. Miller C, Savoie FH. Glenohumeral abnormalities associated with full-thickness tears of the rotator cuff. Orthop Rev 1994;23:159–162

22. Gardner MJ, Griffith MH, Dines JS et al. The extended anterolateral acromial approach allows minimally invasive access to the proximal humerus. Clin Orthop Relat Res 2005;434:123–129

23. St. Pierre P, Olson EJ, Elliott JJ et al. Tendon healing to cortical bone compared with healing to cancellous trough. A biochemical and histological evaluation in goats. J Bone Joint Surg 1995;77:1858–1866

24. Ma CB, Comerford L, Wilson J et al. Biomechanical evaluation of arthroscopic rotator cuff repairs: double-row compared with single-row fixation. J Bone Joint Surg Am 2006;88(2):403–410

25. Fealy S, Kingham TP, Altchek DW. Mini-open RTC repair using a two-row fixation technique: outcomes analysis in patients with small, moderate, and large rotator cuff tears. Arthroscopy 2002;18:665–670

26. Bungaro P, Rotini R, Traina F et al. Comparative and experimental study on different tendinous grasping techniques in rotator cuff repair: a new reinforced stitch. Chir Organi Mov 2005;90(2):113–119

27. Paulos LE, Kody MH. Arthroscopically enhanced "miniapproach" to rotator cuff repair: preliminary results. Arthroscopy 1990;6:55–60

28. Liu SH. Arthroscopically assisted rotator cuff repair. J Bone Joint Surg Br 1994;76:592–595

29. Blevins FT, Warren RF, Cavo C, Altchek DW, Dines D, Palletta G, Wickiewicz TL. Arthroscopic assisted rotator cuff repair: results using a mini-open deltoid splitting approach. Arthroscopy 1996;12:50–59

30. Werner JJ, Goitz RJ, Irrgang JJ et al. Arthroscopic-assisted rotator cuff repair: patient selection and treatment outcome. J Shoulder Elbow Surg 1997;6:463–472

31. Pollock RG, Flatow EL. The rotator cuff: full-thickness tears: mini-open repair. Orthop Clin North Am 1997;28:169–177

32. Park JY, Levine WN, Marra G et al. Portal-extension approach for the repair of small and medium rotator cuff tears. Am J Sports Med 2000;28:312–316

33. Hersch JC, Sgaglione NA. Arthroscopically assisted mini-open rotator cuff repairs: functional outcome at two- to seven-year follow-up. Am J Sports Med 2000;28:301–311

34. Shinners TJ, Noordsij PG, Orwin JF. Arthroscopically assisted mini-open rotator cuff repair. Arthroscopy 2002;18:21–26

35. Posada A, Uribe JW, Hechtman KS et al. Mini-deltoid splitting rotator cuff repair. Do results deteriorate with time? Arthroscopy 2000;16:137–141

36. Zandi H, Coghlan JA, Bell SN. Mini-incision rotator cuff repair: a longitudinal assessment with no deterioration of result up to 9 years. J Shoulder Elbow Surg 2006;15:135–139

37. Baker CL, Liu SH. Comparison of open and arthroscopically assisted rotator cuff repairs. Am J Sports Med 1995;23:99–104

38. Weber SC, Schaefer R. "Mini-open" versus traditional open repair in the management of small and moderate size tears of the rotator cuff. Arthroscopy 1993;9:365–366

39. Hata Y, Saitoh S, Murakami N et al. A less invasive surgery for rotator cuff tear: mini-open repair. J Shoulder Elbow Surg 2001;10:11–16

40. Ide J, Maeda S, Takagi K. A comparison of arthroscopic and open rotator cuff repair. Arthroscopy 2005;21: 1090–1098

41. Buess E, Steuber K, Waibl B. Open versus arthroscopic rotator cuff repair: a comparative view of 96 cases. Arthroscopy 2005;21:597–604

42. Sauerbrey AM, Getz CL, Piancastelli M et al. Arthroscopic versus mini-open rotator cuff repair: a comparison of clinical outcome. Arthroscopy 2005;21:1415–1420

43. Verma NN, Dunn W, Adler RS et al. All-arthroscopic versus mini-open rotator cuff repair: a retrospective review with minimum 2-year follow-up. Arthroscopy 2006;22:587–594

44. Youm T, Murray DH, Kubiak EN et al. Arthroscopic versus mini-open rotator cuff repair: a comparison of clinical outcomes and patient satisfaction. J Shoulder Elbow Surg 2005;14:455–459

45. Macdermid JC, Holtby R, Razmjou H et al. All-arthroscopic versus mini-open repair of small or moderate-sized rotator cuff tears: a protocol for a randomized trial. BMC Musculoskelet Disord 2006; 7:11

Minimally Invasive Treatment of Greater Tuberosity Fractures

5

Brian Magovern, Xavier Duralde, and Guido Marra

The proximal humerus tends to fracture into four distinct fragments: the humeral shaft, the greater and lesser tuberosities, and the articular surface [1]. Neer based his classification system on displacement of these fragments by greater than 1 cm or angulation of more than 45°. In a retrospective review, Neer found that 85% of fractures were considered to be minimally displaced and nonoperative management led to satisfactory results. Displaced two-part greater tuberosity fractures, according to the above criteria, were treated with open reduction and internal fixation [1, 2].

Several authors, however, have advocated treatment that is more aggressive for fractures of the greater tuberosity. Five millimeters of displacement, particularly in the superior direction, has been suggested as an indication for operative management [3–5]. The major deforming forces on the greater tuberosity are the supraspinatus, infraspinatus, and teres minor, resulting in superior and/or posterior pull of the fragment. Malunion with superior displacement may lead to painful impingement and posterior displacement may result in loss of external rotation, which can be challenging to treat [6–8].

Minimally invasive techniques have become increasingly popular in the field of orthopedic surgery. Examples include two-incision total hip arthroplasty [9] and minimally invasive lumbar

disc excision [10]. A great deal of recent research has focused on minimally invasive fracture care such as submuscular plating of long bone fractures [11–15]. When compared with conventional methods, the limited soft tissue and periosteal disruption with less invasive techniques may increase healing rates, speed recovery, and improve cosmesis. While a deltopectoral approach is most often utilized for open reduction of more complex proximal humerus fractures, several less invasive methods have been described for treatment of isolated greater tuberosity fractures. These include arthroscopic treatment [16–21], percutaneous pinning [22], and open reduction through a superior deltoid-splitting approach [5, 7, 23, 24], which will be discussed below.

Preoperative Planning/Imaging

Isolated fractures of the greater tuberosity are relatively uncommon [7] and they are frequently overlooked [25]. Up to 15% occur in association with glenohumeral dislocation [19] (Fig. 5.1) and a careful neurovascular exam is essential in the preoperative evaluation. Many patients who sustain proximal humerus fractures are elderly and have significant medical comorbidities. A proper medical evaluation should be considered as part of the standard preoperative plan.

A complete series of radiographs including anteroposterior (AP), outlet, and axillary views should be obtained (Figs. 5.2–5.4). If the patient is unable to tolerate positioning for an axillary

B. Magovern (✉)
Harbor-UCLA Medical Center, Private Practice,
Orthopaedic Institute, Torrance, CA, USA
e-mail: magovernb@hotmail.com

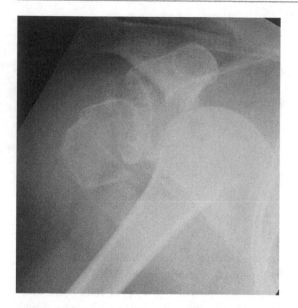

Fig. 5.1 Glenohumeral dislocation with a greater tuberosity fracture

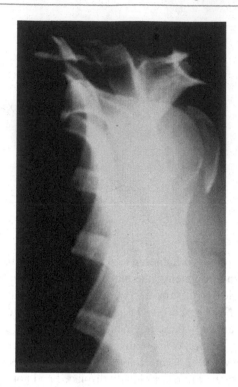

Fig. 5.3 Outlet view

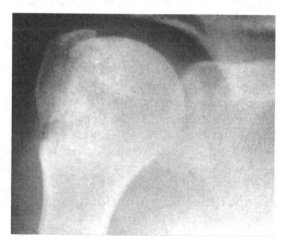

Fig. 5.2 AP view, note superior displacement

view, a Velpeau radiograph may substitute. Rotational AP views may add additional information in determining displacement [26]. Numerous studies have documented poor interobserver and intraobserver reliability in the classification of proximal humerus fractures [27–29], and identifying the degree of displacement of greater tuberosity fractures can be challenging. Posterior displacement of the greater tuberosity may be masked by the humeral head on the AP view and

is best visualized on the axillary view [30]. Superior displacement of the greater tuberosity, on the other hand, is best appreciated on the AP view in external rotation [26]. A recent cadaveric study found significant agreement in regard to treatment recommendations of fractures of the greater tuberosity after review of a series of four standard radiographs (AP in internal and external rotation, outlet, and axillary views) [26].

The use of computed tomography (CT) may increase the reliability of fracture classification and help to determine optimal management (Fig. 5.5) [29]. Other authors, however, have found CT to offer little in the evaluation and treatment of greater tuberosity fractures [31]. In all cases, high-quality radiographs must be obtained and scrutinized prior to making decisions regarding further imaging and subsequent treatment. With minimally invasive techniques of fixation, direct visualization of the reduction may be limited, and intraoperative fluoroscopy should be considered to confirm anatomic reduction.

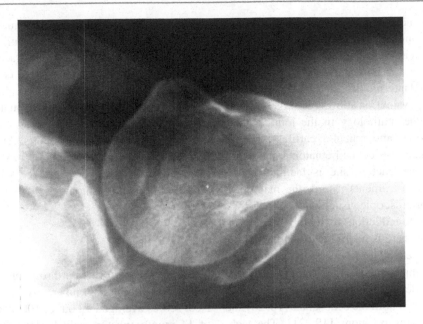

Fig. 5.4   Axillary view, note posterior displacement

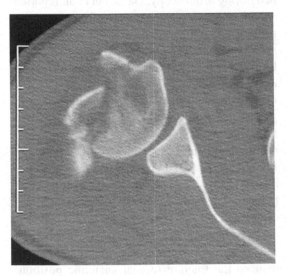

Fig. 5.5   CT scan of a greater tuberosity fracture

Operative Treatment of Displaced Greater Tuberosity Fractures

Arthroscopic Repair of Greater Tuberosity Fractures

Shoulder arthroscopy affords excellent visualization of the glenohumeral joint and subacromial space with less morbidity than conventional open techniques. Arthroscopy has become widely accepted as a valuable and viable option in the management of a broad spectrum of shoulder pathology [32–34]. Similar to reports of arthroscopic treatment of distal radius and tibial plateau fractures [35, 36], shoulder arthroscopy may assist in the evaluation and management of fractures of the shoulder region [16–21, 37–39]. Schai et al. performed diagnostic arthroscopy on 80 patients with shoulder girdle fractures. The authors identified a large percentage of secondary soft tissue lesions, such as labral tears, which may not have been visualized with conventional radiographic techniques [37]. Carro et al. reported an excellent outcome in a patient with a glenoid rim fracture treated with percutaneous pinning under arthroscopic visualization [38]. Kim et al. performed arthroscopy on 23 patients who had persistent pain 6 months after sustaining minimally displaced fractures of the greater tuberosity. Partial-thickness rotator cuff tears were found in all patients [39].

Arthroscopic fixation of greater tuberosity fractures was first reported by Geissler et al. in 1994 [16]. Since then, reports of arthroscopic treatment of greater tuberosity fractures have become more frequent [18–21]. Patients considered for this procedure must have adequate bone stock and a noncomminuted fragment that will support fixation with two or three screws.

Bonsell et al. reported four major advantages of arthroscopic treatment over traditional open reduction and internal fixation (ORIF) [19]. First, arthroscopic evaluation allows the surgeon visual access to other pathology in the joint, namely Bankart lesions and articular cartilage defects. Second, evacuation of the hematoma and debridement of the fracture site is facilitated with arthroscopic instruments. Third, the magnification under arthroscopic visualization allows for a more anatomic reduction of the tuberosity fragment. Lastly, there is no dissection of the deltoid muscle, theoretically decreasing the risk of axillary nerve injury and hastening postoperative recovery of deltoid function. The procedure has been reported in both the beachchair [18, 20] and lateral decubitus positions [19, 21]. The technique as described by Taverna et al. is outlined below [20].

Technique

The initial posterior viewing portal is made slightly more superior and lateral than that used classically (0.5 cm medial and 0.5 cm inferior to the posterolateral edge of the acromion). An anterior portal is created and a diagnostic evaluation of the glenohumeral joint is performed. Repair of any identified labral injuries, or other soft tissue pathology, is carried out at this time. The subacromial space is now examined and a lateral portal is created with spinal needle localization. Once the fracture has been identified and remaining hematoma has been thoroughly evacuated, the fracture bed is debrided of all fibrous tissue with a shaver and the surface is abraded with an arthroscopic burr. A blunt trocar placed through the lateral portal is used to reduce the fracture by pushing the tuberosity fragment anteriorly and inferiorly. Alternatively, a grasper placed from the anterior portal can be used to pull the cuff tendon attached to the fracture fragment in order to reduce the fracture into an anatomic position. Once reduction is obtained and confirmed fluoroscopically, two Kirschner wires are introduced percutaneously under arthroscopic guidance until they reach subchondral bone. Cannulated screws with or without a washer are then placed over the guide wires and advanced until compression across the fracture site is obtained. Again, fluoroscopy is used to evaluate the quality of the reduction. The diameter of the screws varies from 3.5 to 7.0 mm in different reports. Arthroscopic visualization confirms that the screws have not penetrated the articular surface. Wounds are closed in standard fashion.

Results

Geissler et al. performed arthroscopic fixation in 14 patients with greater tuberosity fractures [16]. Neer scores averaged 92 out of 100 at an average of 14 months postoperatively. Of note, 93% of patients had secondary soft tissue lesions identified during arthroscopy. Gartsman et al. reported on the arthroscopic treatment of an acute traumatic anterior glenohumeral dislocation with an associated greater tuberosity fracture [18]. Intraoperatively, the author performed a Bankart repair followed by fixation of the greater tuberosity fracture with one 7.0-mm cannulated screw. At the 2-year follow-up, the patient had regained full range of motion and strength, had no pain, and had radiographic evidence of fracture union. Bonsell and Buford described arthroscopic reduction and fixation of a greater tuberosity fracture in the lateral decubitus position using two 4.5-mm cannulated screws [19]. The authors noted that one advantage of the lateral decubitus position was that placement of the arm in abduction reduced the fracture to near anatomic position. The patient began pendulum exercises in the immediate postoperative period and by 2 months had complete range of motion and no limitations in his activities. The entire procedure was performed without entering the subacromial space. Taverna et al. reported that they have treated patients with this technique since 1997 and have had "remarkable clinical results" [19].

Although no controlled studies exist, these results are promising. Arthroscopic assistance and fixation of greater tuberosity fractures may

Fig. 5.6 Superior
deltoid-splitting approach

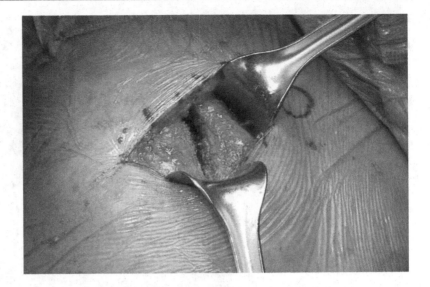

decrease the morbidity associated with open techniques leading to a faster recovery, decreased pain, and improved cosmesis. Arthroscopy also allows the simultaneous management of associated pathology. The procedure, however, can be technically demanding with a steep learning curve, and not all greater tuberosity fractures are amenable to arthroscopic fixation. An anatomic reduction should not be sacrificed in order to perform a less invasive technique. The procedure must be converted to an open reduction if the fracture cannot be reduced anatomically by arthroscopic means [18–21].

Percutaneous Fixation

Closed reduction and percutaneous pinning of proximal humerus fractures is a reliable means for stable fixation in certain patients [22, 23, 40]. Although it is less rigid biomechanically than plate and screw constructs [41], percutaneous pinning may be used in patients with good bone quality and noncomminuted fracture fragments [23]. It is essential that an acceptable reduction can be obtained by closed means. Percutaneous methods of fixation posses a major advantage over open reduction and internal fixation in that there is essentially no soft tissue dissection and minimal risk of iatrogenic avascular necrosis.

Percutaneous fixation of isolated greater tuberosity fractures has rarely been reported. Chen et al. treated 19 patients with proximal humerus fractures percutaneously [22]. Two patients had isolated greater tuberosity fractures treated with a combination of percutaneous pins and screws. Both patients had excellent outcomes according to the criteria of Neer at an average of 28 months postoperatively [22]. Achieving reduction of a displaced greater tuberosity may be challenging via percutaneous methods secondary to the deforming forces contributed by the rotator cuff. If a closed reduction cannot be obtained and an open reduction is necessary, pins may be used for fixation once reduction is achieved. The pins are then placed in a manner similar to that used for more complex proximal humerus fractures.

Superior Deltoid-Splitting Approach

For the majority of displaced proximal humerus fractures, a deltopectoral approach provides the best access for open reduction. Fractures of the greater tuberosity are unique in that exposure may be gained by a superior deltoid-splitting approach (Fig. 5.6). In fact, this limited incision and dissection yields better visualization and allows improved manipulation and fixation of the fracture than a deltopectoral incision [7]. A lateral

Fig. 5.7 Grasping sutures are used to manipulate the fracture fragment

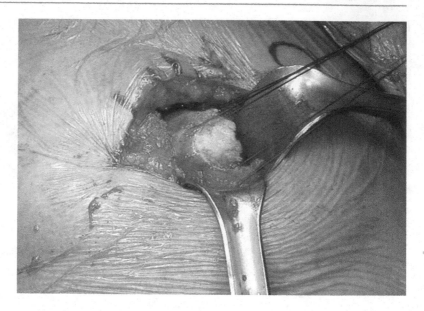

exposure may also decrease the risk of avascular necrosis, as there is less dissection near the bicipital groove [42]. In complex proximal humerus fractures, a two-incision technique has been proposed that uses the lateral approach for reduction of the tuberosity and a second deltopectoral approach for the remaining fragments [43].

Surgical Approach

A 4- to 5-cm incision is made in Langer's lines off the lateral border of the acromion [7, 24]. The superficial fat is bluntly dissected from the deltoid fascia. A longitudinal split is made in the deltoid fascia in line with the muscle fibers at the anterolateral border of the acromion. Alternatively, the split may be made more posteriorly depending on the size and degree of displacement of the greater tuberosity fragment. The biggest risk of this exposure is damage to branches of the axillary nerve, which have been reported to lie 3–5 cm distal to the anterolateral acromion [44, 45]. A stay suture may be placed at the inferior extent of the deltoid in an effort to protect the nerve if preferred. Great care is taken not to disrupt the deltoid origin from the acromion. If necessary,

this approach may be extended by axillary nerve dissection distally [46].

Several grasping sutures are placed in the tuberosity fragment or adjacent cuff tissue to allow safe manipulation of the fragment (Fig. 5.7). Once the fragment is mobilized and reduced, several options exist for fixation, depending on bone quality, degree of comminution, and size of the fragment. These include screws [47, 48], wires, and sutures [7]. Stable anatomic fixation of displaced greater tuberosity fractures is challenged by the deforming forces of the intact rotator cuff and the poor bone quality of the tuberosity [49]. In older patients, the tuberosities may consist of little more than an eggshell of cortical bone with very small amounts of cancellous bone inside and are often inadequate for screw fixation [49, 50]. The strongest structure in the area may be the rotator cuff tendon itself and stable fixation requires utilization of the rotator cuff [7, 24].

Fixation with heavy nonabsorbable suture has been reported with excellent results [7, 24]. The sutures are placed through multiple drill holes through bone adjacent to the fracture bed. In the section below, a two-layered suture repair utilizing suture anchors and cerclage sutures is described.

Fig. 5.8 (a, b)
Overreduction of the
fracture fragment

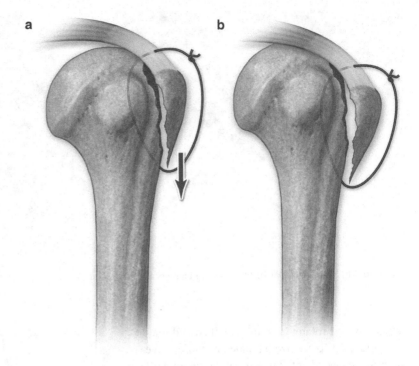

Suture Anchor Technique

Traditional techniques for repair of displaced two-part greater tuberosity fractures advocate a suture technique similar to rotator cuff repair utilizing cerclage braided nonabsorbable sutures. This technique runs the risk of over reduction of the greater tuberosity as tightening of the sutures will advance the greater tuberosity distally until the inferior edge of the greater tuberosity fragment comes into contact with the drill hole placed distally at the humeral shaft (Figs. 5.8 and 5.9). This displacement will be even greater if comminution is encountered in the tuberosity fragment allowing greater displacement of the tuberosity inferiorly and nonanatomic reduction of the rotator cuff relative to the humeral head.

This technique has been utilized in rotator cuff repair to obtain greater contact between the cuff tissue and tuberosity and this slight modification in fracture management allows anatomically precise replacement of the tendon relative to the humeral head along with excellent compression of the tuberosity fragment to obtain adequate bony healing [24].

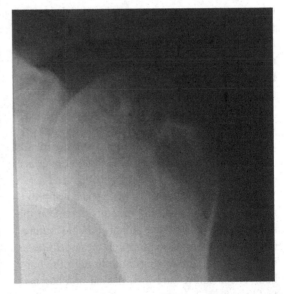

Fig. 5.9 AP X-ray demonstrates healing in an over reduced position

The superior deltoid-splitting approach is utilized to expose the displaced greater tuberosity fracture and may or may not be combined with acromioplasty depending on acromial morphology and concomitant rotator cuff disease. The greater

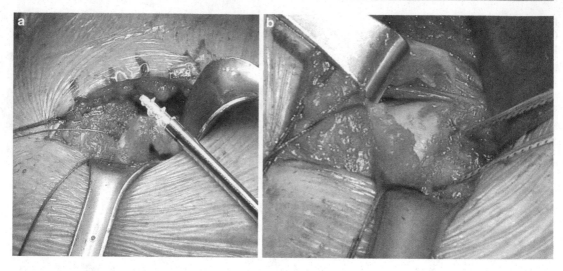

Fig. 5.10 (a) Suture anchor. (b) Placement of anchors at the articular margin

tuberosity and rotator cuff are identified and traction sutures utilizing size 0 braided nonabsorbable sutures are placed at the margin of the rotator cuff at the junction with the greater tuberosity. The tuberosity fragment is assessed and debrided of fracture hematoma. No bone is debrided. The bed for the greater tuberosity is similarly prepared. A row of suture anchors is then placed at the junction between the bony bed of the greater tuberosity on the humerus and the articular margin (Fig. 5.10). These are placed at 45° or the "dead man's angle" into the humeral head. The sutures through the suture anchors are then passed through the rotator cuff tendons directly at the bone-tendon interface on the greater tuberosity fragment (Fig. 5.11).

A row of drill holes is then placed approximately 1 cm distal to the osseous defect on the humeral shaft. Braided nonabsorbable sutures (size 5) are then passed through these drill holes in the distal humeral shaft and through the bony bed. These sutures are then passed in a cerclage fashion through the rotator cuff tendon again at the junction of the bone-tendon interface. The suture anchor sutures are tied first, ensuring anatomic repositioning of the rotator cuff relative to the humeral head. If a significant bony defect is noted, morselized cancellous bone graft with demineralized bone matrix can be inserted into

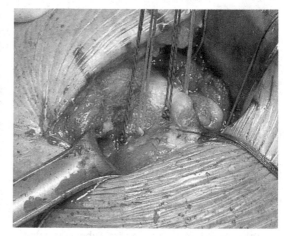

Fig. 5.11 Sutures from the anchors are placed through rotator cuff tendon and tied down

the greater tuberosity bed. The cerclage sutures are then tied over the greater tuberosity fragment to close this fragment as a book and create compression across the fragment (Figs. 5.12–5.14). Tying of the suture anchor sutures first ensures that over reduction of the greater tuberosity cannot occur. Secure closure of the deltoid is then performed using size 0 nonabsorbable braided sutures. Suction drainage is utilized if significant bleeding is noted.

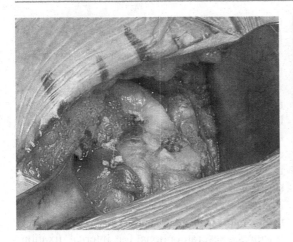

Fig. 5.12 Cerclage sutures are passed around the fragment and tied down to obtain compression across the fracture

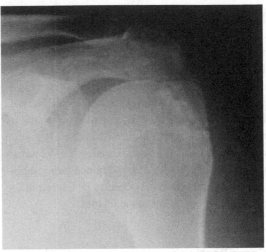

Fig. 5.14 Reduction of the tuberosity fracture in an anatomic position

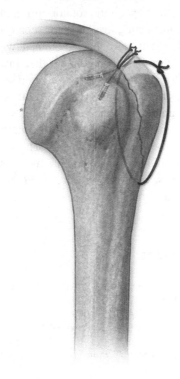

Fig. 5.13 Diagram demonstrates suture construct

Results

Few reports are dedicated solely to the management of isolated greater tuberosity fractures. Many studies group the treatment and outcomes of isolated tuberosity fractures along with more complex three- and four-part proximal humerus fractures, sometimes making outcomes difficult to discern from the literature. Flatow et al. treated 12 patients with greater tuberosity fractures using a superior deltoid-splitting approach and heavy nonabsorbable suture fixation [7]. Outcomes were excellent in all 12 of the patients at an average of 5-year follow-up. All fractures healed radiographically without loss of reduction. Active elevation and external rotation averaged 170° and 63°, respectively. Patients were able to reach behind their back, on average, to the ninth thoracic vertebra. Park et al. obtained 89% good to excellent results in a series of 27 patients with two- and three-part proximal humerus fractures treated in a manner similar to Flatow's series [24]. Although the authors did not separately list the outcomes of the two-part greater tuberosity group, they noted that there was no significant difference between different fracture types. Chun et al. reported the outcome of 137 patients with proximal humerus fractures [48]. Twenty-four patients had greater tuberosity fractures, of which, ten were treated with open reduction and internal fixation. Eight of these were treated with screw fixation. Although 8 of 11 patients had a satisfactory result, the authors did not evaluate the patients separately based on whether they received conservative or operative treatment.

Postoperative Management

Patients are placed in a sling postoperatively. Passive range of motion is instituted on postoperative day one within safe limits determined intraoperatively. These passive exercises are performed for the first 6 weeks, at which time patients are advanced to active-assisted exercises. Resistive exercises are added at approximately 10–12 weeks once bony healing has been obtained radiographically. Rehabilitation may need to be altered in the presence of other soft tissue lesions.

Complications

Complications specific to operative treatment of greater tuberosity fractures are infrequently reported in the literature. As with any surgery, infection, bleeding, and anesthetic-related complications can occur. One patient in Flatow's series sustained an axillary nerve palsy postoperatively [7]. It had completely resolved by 9 months and the patient had a good result. One patient in Park's series required arthroscopic lysis of adhesions 6 months postoperatively for adhesive capsulitis and ultimately ended up with an unsatisfactory result [24]. Obtaining an anatomic reduction and protecting the axillary nerve are two important ways to avoid complications and achieve optimal results.

Summary

Displaced fractures of the greater tuberosity may result in significant disability if not evaluated and treated appropriately. Even with modern imaging techniques, proper identification and classification of fractures can be challenging. The indication for operative repair of greater tuberosity fractures has been more aggressive than it has with other fractures of the proximal humerus. With the increased popularity of minimally invasive surgery, techniques that limit soft tissue dissection and potentially hasten recovery are becoming more attractive. Fractures of the greater tuberosity are unique in that several less invasive methods of fixation are available.

Arthroscopic and arthroscopic-assisted fixation techniques are being reported more frequently with promising clinical results. If a satisfactory reduction cannot be achieved, the procedure must be converted to an open reduction. Closed reduction and percutaneous pinning is an option, although rarely used for isolated greater tuberosity fractures. If open reduction is preferred, a superior deltoid-splitting approach offers excellent exposure and is less invasive than the deltopectoral approach used for most proximal humerus fractures. Several options for internal fixation exist, including screws and heavy sutures. Patient factors, such as poor bone stock or fracture fragmentation, may preclude the use of screw fixation. In these cases, the rotator cuff tendon is the strongest structure available for repair. Excellent clinical results have been obtained with suture fixation through bone tunnels that incorporates the rotator cuff tendon. A two-layered suture technique using suture anchors, as outlined above, allows anatomic placement and secure compressive fixation of the tendon and tuberosity fragment on the humeral head. The goal of the above techniques, identical to more traditional approaches, is stable internal fixation to allow early motion.

References

1. Neer CS II. Displaced Proximal Humeral Fractures. Part I. Classification and Evaluation. *J Bone Joint Surg* 1970;52-A:1077–1089
2. Neer CS II. Displaced Proximal Humeral Fractures. Part II. Treatment of Three-Part and Four-Part Displacement. *J Bone Joint Surg* 1970;52-A: 1090–1103
3. McLaughlin HL. Dislocation of the Shoulder with Tuberosity Fracture. *Surg Clin North Am* 1963;43: 1615–1620
4. Levy AS. Greater Tuberosity Fractures of the Humerus. *Orthop Trans* 1998;22:594
5. Green A, Izzi J. Isolated Fractures of the Greater Tuberosity of the Proximal Humerus. *J Shoulder Elbow Surg* 2003;12:641–649
6. Hawkins RJ, Angelo RL. Displaced Proximal Humeral Fractures. Selecting Treatment, Avoiding Pitfalls. *Orthop Clin North Am* 1987;18:421–431

7. Flatow EL, Cuomo F, Maday MG, et al. Open Reduction and Internal Fixation of Two-Part Displaced Fractures of the Greater Tuberosity of the Proximal Part of the Humerus. *J Bone Joint Surg* 1991; 73-A:1213–1218

8. Berdjiklian PK, Iannotti JP, Norris TR, et al. Operative Treatment of Malunion of a Fracture of the Proximal Aspect of the Humerus. *J Bone Joint Surg* 1998;80A:1484–1497

9. Berger RA. Total Hip Arthroplasty Using the Minimally Invasive Two-Incision Approach. *Clin Orthop Relat Res* 2003;417:232–241

10. Yeung AT, Tsou PT. Posterolateral Endoscopic Excision for Lumbar Disc Herniation: Surgical Technique, Outcome, and Complications in 307 Consecutive Cases. *Spine* 2002;27:722–731

11. Collinge CA, Sanders RW. Percutaneous Plating in the Lower Extremity. *J Am Acad Orthop Surg* 2000;8:211–216

12. Schandelmaier P, Partenheimer A, Koenemann B, et al. Distal Femoral Fractures and LISS Stabilization. *Injury* 2001;32 (S3): SC55–SC63

13. Fankhauser F, Gruber G, Schippinger G, et al. Minimal-invasive Treatment of Distal Femoral Fractures with the LISS (Less Invasive Stabilization System): A Prospective Study of 30 Fractures with a Follow up of 20 Months. *Acta Orthop Scand* 2004;75:56–60

14. Anglen J, Choi L. Treatment Options in Pediatric Femoral Shaft Fractures. *J Orthop Trauma* 2005;19: 724–733

15. Boldin C, Fankhauser F, Hofer HP, Szyszkowitz R. Three-Year Results of Proximal Tibia Fractures Treated with the LISS. *Clin Orthop Relat Res* 2006;445:222–229

16. Geissler WB, Petrie SG, Savoie FH. Arthroscopic Fixation of Greater Tuberosity Fractures of the Humerus (Abstract). *Arthroscopy* 1994;10:344

17. Gartsman GM, Taverna E. Arthroscopic Treatment of Rotator Cuff Tear and Greater Tuberosity Fracture Nonunion. *Arthroscopy* 1996;12:242–244

18. Gartsman GM, Taverna E, Hammerman SM. Arthroscopic Treatment of Acute Traumatic Anterior Glenohumeral Dislocation and Greater Tuberosity Fracture. *Arthroscopy* 1999;15:648–650

19. Bonsell S, Buford DA. Arthroscopic Reduction and Internal Fixation of a Greater Tuberosity Fracture of the Shoulder: A Case Report. *J Shoulder Elbow Surg* 2003;12:397–400

20. Taverna E, Sansone V, Battistella F. Arthroscopic Treatment for Greater Tuberosity Fractures: Rationale and Surgical Technique. *Arthroscopy* 2004;20:e53–e57

21. Carrera EF, Matsumoto MH, Netto NA, Faloppa F. Fixation of Greater Tuberosity Fractures. *Arthroscopy* 2004;20:e109–e111

22. Chen C, Chao E, Tu Y, et al. Closed Management and Percutaneous Fixation of Unstable Proximal Humerus Fractures. *J Trauma* 1998;45:1039–1045

23. Williams GR, Wong KL. Two-part and Three-part Fractures: Open Reduction and Internal Fixation Versus Closed Reduction and Percutaneous Pinning. *Orthop Clin North Am* 2000;31:1–21

24. Park MC, Murthi AM, Roth NS, et al. Two-part and Three-part Fractures of the Proximal Humerus Treated with Suture Fixation. *J Orthop Trauma* 2003;17:319–325

25. Ogawa K, Yoshida A, Ikegami H. Isolated Fractures of the Greater Tuberosity of the Humerus: Solutions to Recognizing a Frequently Overlooked Fracture. *J Trauma* 2003;54:713–717

26. Parsons BO, Klepps SJ, Miller S, et al. Reliability and Reproducibility of Radiographs of Greater Tuberosity Displacement. *J Bone Joint Surg* 2005;87A:58–65

27. Sidor ML, Zuckerman JD, Lyon T, et al. The Neer Classification System for Proximal Humeral Fractures. An Assessment of Interobserver Reliability and Intraobserver Reproducibility. *J Bone Joint Surg* 1993;75A:1745–1750

28. Siebenrock KA, Gerber C. The Reproducibility of Classification of Fractures of the Proximal End of the Humerus. *J Bone Joint Surg* 1993;75A:1751–1755

29. Bernstein J, Adler L, Blank JE, et al. Evaluation of the Neer System of Classification of Proximal Humeral Fractures with Computerized Tomographic Scans and Plain Radiographs. *J Bone Joint Surg* 1996;78A: 1371–1375

30. Blaine TA, Bigliani LU, Levine WN. Fractures of the Proximal Humerus. In: Rockwood CA, et al (eds.) *The Shoulder*. Philadelphia: Saunders, 2004, pp. 355–412

31. Sjoden GO, Movin T, Guntner P, et al. Poor Reproducibility of Classification of Proximal Humerus Fractures. Additional CT of Minor Value. *Acta Orthop Scand* 1997;68:239–242

32. Burkhart SS, Lo IKY. Arthroscopic Rotator Cuff Repair. *J Am Acad Orthop Surg* 2006;14:333–346

33. Kim S, Ha K, Kim S. Bankart Repair in Traumatic Anterior Shoulder Instability: Open Versus Arthroscopic Technique. *Arthroscopy* 2002;18: 755–763

34. Nam EK, Snyder SJ. The Diagnosis and Treatment of Superior Labrum, Anterior and Posterior (SLAP) Lesion. *Am J Sports Med* 2003;31:798–810

35. Lubowitz JH, Elson WS, Guttmann D. Part I: Arthroscopic Management of Tibial Plateau Fractures. *Arthroscopy* 2004;20:1063–1070

36. Ruch DS, Vallee J, Poehling GG, et al. Arthroscopic Reduction Versus Fluoroscopic Reduction in the Management in the Management of Intra-articular Distal Radius Fractures. *Arthroscopy* 2004;20: 225–230

37. Schai PA, Hintermann B, Koris MJ. Preoperative Arthroscopic Assessment of Fractures About the Shoulder. *Arthroscopy* 1999;15:827–835

38. Carro LP, Nunez MP, Llata JIE. Arthroscopic-Assisted Reduction and Percutaneous External Fixation of a Displaced Intra-articular Glenoid Fracture. *Arthroscopy* 1999;15:211–214

39. Kim S, Ha K. Arthroscopic Treatment of Symptomatic Shoulders with Minimally Displaced Greater Tuberosity Fracture. *Arthroscopy* 2000;16:695–700

40. Jaberg H, Warner JJP, Jakob RP. Percutaneous Stabilization of Unstable Fractures of the Humerus. *J Bone Joint Surg* 1992;74-A:508–515

41. Naidu SH, Bixler B, Capo JT, et al. Percutaneous Pinning of Proximal Humerus Fractures: A Biomechanical Study. *Orthopaedics* 1997;20: 1073–1076

42. Gerber C, Schneeberger AG, Vinh T. The Arterial Vascularization of the Humeral Head: An Anatomical Study. *J Bone Joint Surg* 1990;72A:1486–1494

43. Gallo RA, Zeiders GJ, Altman GT. Two-Incision Technique for Treatment of Complex Proximal Humerus Fractures. *J Orthop Trauma* 2005;19:734–740

44. Burkhead WZ, Scheinberg RR, Box G. Surgical Anatomy of the Axillary Nerve. *J Shoulder Elbow Surg* 1992;1:31–36

45. Hoppenfeld S, de Boer P. The Shoulder, In: Hoppenfeld S, de Boer P (eds.) *Surgical Exposures in Orthopaedics: The Anatomic Approach*. Philadelphia: Lippincott, 1994, pp. 1–50

46. Gardner MJ, Griffith MH, Dines JS, et al. The Extended Anterolateral Acromial Approach Allows Minimally Invasive Access to the Proximal Humerus. *Clin Orthop Relat Res* 2005;434:123–129

47. Paavolainen P, Bjorkenheim J, Slatis P, Paukku P. Operative Treatment of Severe Proximal Humeral Fractures. *Acta Orthop Scand* 1983;54:374–379

48. Chun J, Groh GI, Rockwood CA. Two-Part Fractures of the Proximal Humerus. *J Shoulder Elbow Surg* 1994;3:273–287

49. Hawkins RJ, Kiefer GN. Internal Fixation Techniques for Proximal Humeral Fractures. *Clin Orthop Relat Res* 1987;223:77–85

50. Earwaker J. Isolated Avulsion Fracture of the Lesser Tuberosity of the Humerus. *Skeletal Radiol* 1990;19: 121–125

Mini-Incision Fixation of Proximal Humeral Four-Part Fractures*

6

Jim C. Hsu and Leesa M. Galatz

Proximal humerus fractures are notoriously difficult to treat. The surrounding rotator cuff musculature makes intraoperative assessment of the reduction of fractures, especially those involving the articular surface, difficult to assess. Even fractures fixed with open reduction and internal fixation often require intraoperative fluoroscopic guidance to ensure appropriate anatomic reduction. The anatomic relationship between the articular surface and the surrounding rotator cuff has a critical influence on the final result. Furthermore, fixation is a challenge to maintain as the rotator cuff exerts strong deforming forces on the tuberosities, which are often of poor bone quality and do not hold hardware well. In spite of this, many unstable proximal humerus fractures are treated successfully with established methods of open reduction and internal fixation.

Four-part proximal humerus fractures, as classified by Neer [1, 2], are particularly problematic. Historically, they have a very high rate of avascular necrosis following fixation. Because of this, Neer recommended hemiarthroplasty for the treatment of these fractures. However, a subgroup of four-part

proximal humerus fractures, the *four-part valgus-impacted fracture*, is readily amenable to reduction and fixation. Neer did not specify this fracture in his initial classification system. In the more recent AO/ASIS classification, however, the valgus-impacted humeral head fracture is regarded as a separate type of fracture [3]. The valgus-impacted four-part fracture is an ideal fracture for minimally invasive fixation, and it is the focus of this chapter.

There has been a surge of interest in minimally invasive techniques in many different subspecialty areas of orthopedics. The recent trauma literature contains several reports of percutaneous fixation of femur, tibia, and tibial pilon fractures [4–6]. Principles of preserving blood supply and minimizing soft tissue stripping are receiving increased attention in fracture fixation. With respect to the treatment of proximal humerus fractures, there have been a few reports in the past several years of successful percutaneous reduction and fixation [7–9]. In selected fractures, percutaneous pinning allows preservation of the intact soft tissue sleeve and periosteal blood supply while obtaining and maintaining a stable reduction. Other potential advantages include smaller incisions, less dissection, and less scarring. A minimally invasive approach minimizes trauma to the rotator cuff and deltoid, and with experience can decrease operative time. While still a difficult, technically demanding procedure, percutaneous pinning of valgus-impacted four-part proximal humerus fractures shows considerable potential. This chapter discusses the unique characteristics of valgus-impacted fractures and outlines in detail the minimally invasive fixation technique.

*Adapted from Hsu J, Galatz LM, Mini-incision Fixation of Proximal Humeral Four-Part Fractures in Scuderi G, Tria A, Berger R (eds), *MIS Techniques in Orthopedics*, New York, Springer, 2006, with kind permission of Springer Science and Business Media, Inc.

L.M. Galatz (✉)
Department of Orthopaedic Surgery, Washington University School of Medicine, St. Louis, MO, USA
e-mail: galatzlewustl.edu

Historical Perspective

Percutaneous pinning has been used in a variety of subtypes of proximal humerus fractures (Table 6.1). Böhler [10] originally described a method of closed reduction and pinning for the treatment of epiphyseal fractures of the proximal end of the humerus in adolescents. This technique has been modified over the years and applied to treat proximal humerus fractures more commonly seen in the older population. In 1991, Jakob [11] reported on the treatment of 19 valgus-impacted four-part proximal humerus fractures, five of which were treated closed. This is the first description of elevation of the valgus-impacted articular fragment with minimal soft tissue dissection to preserve the remaining blood supply to the proximal humerus. The valgus-impacted four-part fracture configuration became recognized as one in which there was a significantly lower rate of avascular necrosis compared with other four-part fractures. In 1995, Resch [12] reported a series of 22 patients with open reduction and internal fixation of the valgus-impacted proximal humerus fracture, further solidifying the understanding of the fracture as one that does not require hemiarthroplasty. In fact, the results of these studies showed better results after fixation than the historical results after hemiarthroplasty.

In 1992, Jaberg et al. [7] reported on percutaneous stabilization of 54 displaced proximal humerus fractures of varying types. In this series, closed reduction was performed and the fractures were stabilized with K wires placed in both antegrade and retrograde fashion. Resch et al. [8] later reported on percutaneous fixation of three- and four-part proximal humerus fractures. The authors described using a pointed hook retractor percutaneously in the subacromial space for reduction of greater tuberosity fragments and elevation of the humeral head in valgus-impacted four-part fractures.

Anatomic Considerations

Four-part valgus-impacted humerus fractures have been described as "impacted with inferior subluxation," [13] "impacted and little displaced fractures," [3] and minimally displaced fractures [14]. Fourteen percent of all humeral head fractures are valgus impacted. The articular segment is impacted into the metaphysis, causing avulsion of both the greater and the lesser tuberosities with a line of fracture through the anatomic neck (Fig. 6.1a, b). The blood supply to the articular segment via the tuberosities is therefore disrupted. The main source of vascularization for the humeral head, the ascending anterolateral branch of the anterior humeral circumflex artery [15, 16], is interrupted at its point of entry into the humeral head in the area of the intertubercular groove. The only remaining blood supply is medially via the periosteum. Numerous vessels ascend along the inferior capsule and periosteum from both the anterior and posterior humeral circumflex arteries to the calcar region of the medial portion of the anatomic neck. Any lateral displacement of the articular fragment damages the periosteal hinge and consequently interrupts this last remaining source of vascularization. Therefore, a true valgus-impacted humeral head fracture will be impacted such that the medial hinge is intact. Any lateral displacement of the head segment has been associated with a higher rate of avascular necrosis [12].

Table 6.1 Fractures amenable to percutaneous pinning

2-part	Surgical neck
	Greater tuberosity
	Lesser tuberosities[a]
3-part	Surgical neck/greater tuberosity
	Surgical neck/lesser tuberosity[a]
4-part	Valgus impacted

[a]Without associated posterior dislocation

Indications for Percutaneous Pinning

Successful outcome after operative treatment of unstable proximal humerus fractures, regardless of approach or choice of hardware, depends on a few critical factors: (1) anatomic reduction,

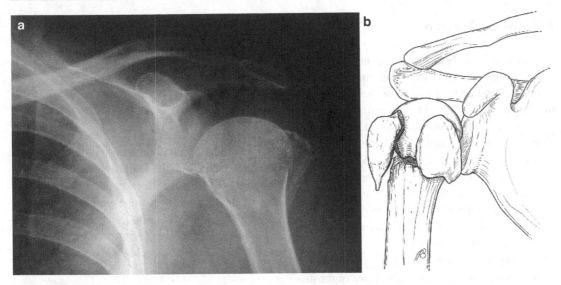

Fig. 6.1 (a) This anteroposterior (AP) radiograph of a valgus-impacted four-part fracture demonstrates the intact medial periosteal hinge with avulsion and lateral displacement of the greater tuberosity. (b) This valgus-impacted four-part fracture drawing also demonstrates the otherwise superimposed lesser tuberosity fragment fracture, making this a true four-part fracture (from Scuderi p. 34)

(2) stable fixation, and (3) careful management of soft tissues. Plate fixation offers a reliably stable construct in patients with good bone quality. The surgical approach and plate application require more extensive soft tissue stripping, which may contribute to the problem of devascularization and subsequent avascular necrosis. Intramedullary rods with cerclage wires are another alternative, and have been shown to be biomechanically stable constructs [17]. However, mechanical impingement in the subacromial space remains a potential problem.

Percutaneous pinning offers an excellent alternative to the open approach in selected fractures (Table 6.2). An anatomic reduction and stable fixation are just as important in this procedure. Patients must have good bone stock to ensure secure pin fixation. The displaced greater tuberosity fragment requiring reduction and fixation must be large and substantial enough to hold one or two screws. An intact medial calcar region is important for stability after reduction of the proximal humerus. This is the portion that must be intact in the valgus-impacted humeral head fracture to preserve the remaining vascularity.

Patient compliance is critical. Therefore, patient selection plays an important role. Postoperative

Table 6.2 Conditions for successful pinning

Good bone stock
Intact medial calcar
Substantial greater tuberosity fragment
Stable reduction under fluoroscopy after pinning
Reliable, cooperative patient

rehabilitation is more conservative than after an open procedure. Patients are generally immobilized for the first couple of weeks. Patients must undergo close surveillance and consistent follow-up in order to prevent complications related to pin migration, either antegrade or retrograde, and to detect any unexpected early loss of fixation.

Percutaneous pinning is contraindicated in (1) patients with poor bone stock, (2) fracture in which there is a comminuted proximal shaft fragment, especially in the medial calcar region, (3) displaced four-part fractures (other than the valgus-impacted configuration) in elderly people requiring hemiarthroplasty, (4) noncompliant patients or patients unable or unwilling to comply with strict follow-up and rehabilitation limitations, and (5) fractures with displaced greater tuberosity fragments that are too comminuted or small for hardware fixation.

Patient Evaluation

Patient evaluation begins with a complete history and physical examination. The mechanism of injury should be noted and all associated injuries thoroughly evaluated. Most proximal humerus fractures are the result of low-energy falls in elderly patients. Another subset of fractures results from high-energy injuries in the younger population. A thorough neurovascular examination should be performed prior to any attempt at percutaneous pinning. The patient's social situation should be assessed in order to discern whether the patient is appropriate in terms of complying with rehabilitation and close follow-up. Patients should be advised that one of the disadvantages of this procedure is that the pins may be uncomfortable in the subcutaneous position. They require subsequent removal as either an office or short operative procedure.

Radiographic evaluation consists of four standard views: an anteroposterior view of the shoulder, an anteroposterior view of the scapula, an axillary view, and a scapular Y. This combination of radiographs is helpful in evaluating posterior displacement of greater tuberosity fragments as well as anterior displacement of the shaft fragment. These X-rays are usually sufficient.

A computed tomography (CT) scan can be considered if further radiographic evaluation is desirable. Three-dimensional reconstructions are rarely necessary. Studies help evaluate the suitability of the particular fracture for percutaneous reduction and fixation.

Elderly people with significant osteopenia and noncompliant patients may be better candidates for open reduction and internal fixation, a procedure that can potentially lead to more secure fixation biomechanically. Less concern exists over loss of fixation and pin migration. Preoperative consent should include possible conversion to an open procedure if the fracture cannot be adequately reduced and held with percutaneous fixation.

Surgical Procedure

Patient Positioning

The patient position must allow unencumbered access to the shoulder, both for easy visualization under fluoroscopy and for pin placement (Fig. 6.2). The patient is placed on a radiolucent operating room table with their head in a head holder such that the shoulder is proximal and lateral to the edge of the table. Adequate visualization of the

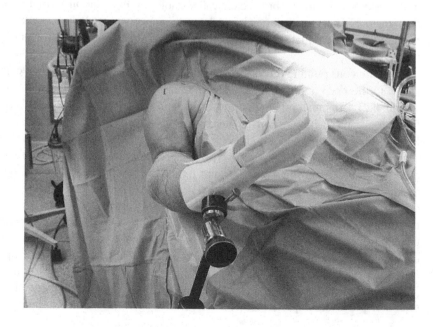

Fig. 6.2 Patient positioning allows for unencumbered access to the anterior, posterior, and lateral shoulder for easy visualization on a radiolucent table as well as pin placement. The reduction portal is drawn in its location approximately 1–2 cm distal to the anterolateral corner of the acromion

shoulder under fluoroscopy should be confirmed before prepping and draping. The procedure can be performed with the patient in the supine position; however, raising the head of the bed 15–20° is often helpful for orientation and instrumentation. A mechanical arm holder is used for positioning the arm during the procedure. The holder can be useful for placing traction on the arm when necessary. The C-arm fluoroscope is positioned at the head of the bed, parallel to the patient, leaving the area lateral to the shoulder open for access and pin placement. Alternatively, the C-arm can be angled perpendicular to the patient; however, it is much more difficult to get an axillary view with the C-arm in this position. The monitor is placed on the opposite side of the patient for easy visualization by the surgeon. We recommend not using an adhesive, plastic drape directly on the skin at the operative site because it can become adherent to the pins inadvertently during insertion and may be introduced into the wound. The shoulder should be draped to accommodate conversion to an open procedure, should it be necessary.

Percutaneous Reduction

Bony landmarks are outlined on the skin, specifically, the acromion, clavicle, and coracoid. A small 1- to 2-cm incision is made 2–3 cm distal to the anterolateral corner of the acromion. Formation of this "reduction portal" facilitates reduction of the fracture percutaneously prior to pin fixation (Fig. 6.3). The reduction portal is positioned distal to the anterolateral corner of the acromion at the level of the surgical neck of the humerus, posterior and lateral to the biceps tendon. The fracture between the greater and the lesser tuberosities lies approximately ½–1 cm posterior to the biceps groove. Localizing the reduction portal over the split between the tuberosities enables elevation of the head fragment by placing the instrument through the natural fracture line.

The deltoid is gently and bluntly spread in order to avoid possible injury to the anterior branch of the axillary nerve in this location. A blunt-tipped elevator or a small bone tamp is

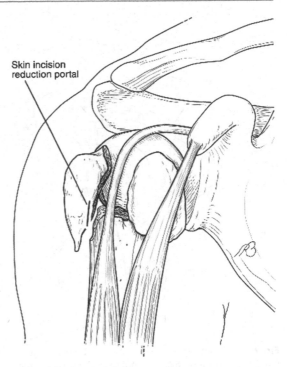

Skin incision
reduction portal

Fig. 6.3 The reduction portal is positioned distal to the anterolateral corner of the acromion at the level of the surgical neck of the humerus. This allows for easy instrumentation between the greater and the lesser tuberosity for reducing the fracture

placed through the *reduction portal* at the level of the surgical neck through the split in the tuberosities and under the lateral aspect of the humeral head (Fig. 6.4). The position is checked under fluoroscopy. The bone tamp or elevator is tapped with a mallet, elevating the head into the reduced position, restoring the normal angle between the humeral shaft and the articular surface of the humeral head. Characteristically, in a valgus-impacted proximal humerus fracture, once the head fragment is reduced anatomically, the tuberosities naturally fall into the reduced position. Occasionally, the lesser tuberosity may still be displaced medially and can potentially require lateral traction via a small hook in the subdeltoid space to bring it into anatomic position. Final reduction is confirmed using fluoroscopic imaging.

A potential pitfall includes overly aggressive impaction with the mallet, leading to loss of cancellous bone in the head fragment and potential

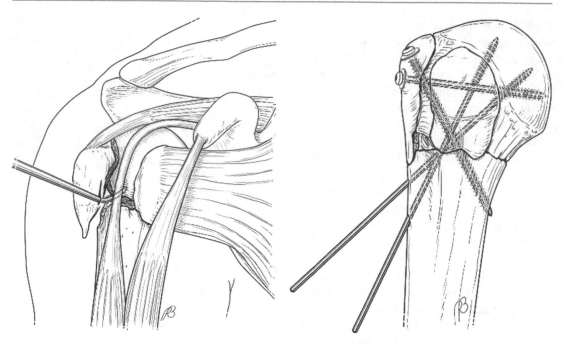

Fig. 6.4 A blunt-tipped elevator or small bone tamp is placed through the reduction portal through the split in the tuberosities and under the lateral aspect of the humeral head in order to elevate the head fragment into an anatomic position

Fig. 6.5 The pins are placed in an anterolateral to posteromedial position because of the anatomic retroversion of the humeral head. Screws should be placed lateral and distal enough to avoid mechanical impingement symptoms in the subacromial space

fracture. Valgus-impacted fractures can only be reduced using this technique before healing has taken place. Ideally, it is recommended in the first 2 weeks after the fracture. Beyond that time, more aggressive manipulation may be required in order to mobilize the head fragment.

Instrumentation

Instrumentation includes 2.5- or 2.7-mm terminally threaded pins. Terminally threaded K wires or, alternatively, guide wires from the Synthes (Synthes, Paoli, PA) 7.3-mm cannulated screw set can be used. Fully threaded pins are not used to protect the soft tissues. Terminal threads are desirable in order to prevent migration. Pins are inserted through very small incisions. Optimally, a drill guide should be used. A drill guide can be obtained from a small fragment fracture set. Alternatively, a drill guide used for arthroscopic anchor insertion can be useful.

Two to three retrograde pins are placed from the shaft into the head fragment. The pins should enter the skin distal to the site where the pins actually enter the bone in order to obtain the correct angle so that the pins do not cut out posteriorly before gaining fixation in the head fragment (Fig. 6.5). The direction of the pins is generally anterolateral to posteromedial because of the anatomic retroversion of the humeral head. Pins should not be placed directly in the coronal plane because of the normal retroversion of the humeral head. This results in pins cutting out anteriorly. The starting points of the pins should not be too close to one another to avoid a stress riser in the lateral cortex. Additionally, the pins should be multidirectional in order to stabilize the construct. Two to three pins parallel to one another will act as a single point of fixation, allowing rotation.

The tuberosities are then secured. Pins or cannulated screws can be used. We prefer fixation with cannulated screws because the ends of the pins protrude through the deltoid and can cause

Fig. 6.6 The pins and screws are placed under fluoroscopic guidance. Reduction of the fracture as well as hardware placement can be checked using continuous fluoroscopy or spot views in multiple positions

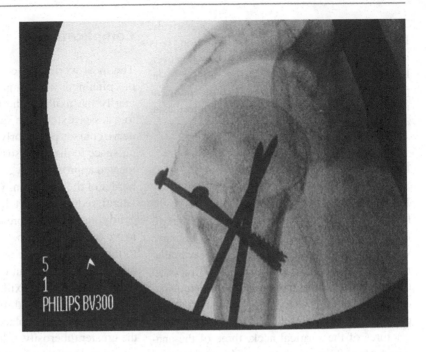

muscle irreparable damage. Pins, if used, must be removed before starting early range-of-motion exercises for this reason. We prefer 4.5-mm cannulated screws to secure the greater tuberosity. The 4.5-mm screws have a substantial guidewire and come in adequate lengths. The guidewire is placed under fluoroscopic guidance through the greater tuberosity approximately 1 cm below the rotator cuff insertion, engaging the medial cortex of the shaft fragment (Fig. 6.6). A screw with a washer is used, but one must be careful not to overtighten the screw because the compression with the washer can potentially fracture the greater tuberosity. Ideally, two screws are placed. The second screw can be a cancellous screw directed into the articular fragment. Often with one antegrade screw and two retrograde pins, there is not enough room in the metaphysis for a second antegrade screw from the greater tuberosity.

Fixation of the lesser tuberosity is debatable. Once the humeral head and greater tuberosity are reduced and fixed, the lesser tuberosity is nearly always in anatomic position. If there is excessive medial displacement, a hook retractor can be used through the reduction portal in the subdeltoid space to move the fragment laterally, and a percutaneous cannulated screw can be placed from the anterior to posterior direction to secure the lesser tuberosity. We generally prefer to leave the lesser tuberosity in the reduced position without additional fixation. It has not been found to result in any functional disability postoperatively.

After percutaneous fixation, the pins are cut below the skin. This reduces the chance of superficial pin tract infection. All of these small incisions are closed using interrupted nylon suture.

Postoperative Management

After the procedure, the affected extremity is immobilized in a sling for approximately 3 weeks. Active wrist, elbow, and hand range-of-motion exercises are encouraged. Radiographs are obtained 1, 3, and 6 weeks postoperatively. If the fracture is thought to be stable, pendulum exercises can be initiated immediately; however, in many cases, pendulum exercises, passive forward flexion in the scapular plane, and external rotation are not started for 3 weeks, provided the fracture remains stable. Active assisted and active range-of-motion exercises are initiated at 6 weeks if there are signs of fracture healing. Progression to light strengthening is as tolerated at that point.

The pins are removed 4–6 weeks postoperatively. In a very unstable fracture configuration, it is optimal to leave the pins in for 6 weeks; however, loosening may necessitate earlier removal. The pins are removed either as an office procedure or in the operating room under local anesthesia, depending on patient and surgeon preference.

Results

Jakob et al. [11] first presented his results of the treatment of 19 valgus-impacted four-part proximal humerus fractures. Five of these fractures were treated closed. He reported an avascular necrosis rate of 26%. Jaberg et al. [7] reported the results of 48 fractures fixed with percutaneous stabilization of unstable fractures of the proximal humerus fracture. This series had 29 fractures of the surgical neck, three of the anatomic neck, 83-part fractures, 54-part fractures, and three fracture dislocations. They had 38 good to excellent results, ten fair, and four poor. One patient with a two-part fracture had avascular necrosis approximately 11 months postoperatively. Eight patients had localized transient avascular necrosis of the small portion of the humeral head that did not necessitate humeral head replacement.

Resch et al. [12] published his results of percutaneous pinning of nine three-part fractures and 18 four-part fractures. None of the three-part fractures went on to avascular necrosis, and all had a good or very good result. There was an 11% incidence of avascular necrosis in the four-part fractures. Those with anatomical reconstructions did very well. Five of these patients had four-part fractures with significant lateral displacement at a humeral head. One of these required revision 1 week after surgery, and one went on to late avascular necrosis. Soete et al. [18] recommended against percutaneous pinning for the treatment of four-part proximal humerus fracture because of avascular necrosis and unsatisfactory reduction. These were not all valgus-impacted proximal humerus fractures, however.

Complications

The most worrisome complication of percutaneous pinning is nerve injury. Nerves at risk are primarily the axillary, the musculocutaneous, and, to a lesser extent, the radial nerve. The axillary nerve courses posteriorly through the quadrangular space to the undersurface of the deltoid and is located approximately 3–5 cm distal to the lateral border of the acromion. When making the anterolateral reduction portal, the deltoid should be gently and bluntly spread in order to avoid any nerve traction. This incision is generally superior to the zone where the nerve is located; however, one should still be cautious during this portion of the procedure. The axillary nerve is also at risk when placing screws through the greater tuberosity. If the screws are placed more inferiorly along the greater tuberosity, a drill guide can be inserted more superiorly and gently advanced distally in order to keep the nerve from the path of the drill.

An anatomic study of percutaneous pinning of the proximal part of the humerus [19] demonstrated that the proximal lateral retrograde pins were located a mean distance of 3 mm from the anterior branch of the axillary nerve. The screws through the tuberosity were located a mean distance of 6 and 7 mm from the axillary nerve and the posterior humeral circumflex artery. While these structures are at risk during placement, they are easily protected if the screws are placed in a careful fashion. The anterior pin is located adjacent to the long head of the biceps tendon, 11 mm from the cephalic vein, and could potentially be near the musculocutaneous nerve [19]. These findings emphasize the importance of using a drill guide. The radial nerve will not be injured as long as the retrograde pins are inserted proximal to the deltoid insertion.

The most common complication is pin migration. Most commonly, the pins back out and become prominent under the skin. Proximal migration into the joint is possible. Percutaneous pinning requires very close follow-up and strict patient compliance. Serious complications of pin migration are prevented by following patients with radiographs at regular intervals. Loss of fixation may occur as with any type of fracture fixation. In some situations, this can be treated with repeat percutaneous pinning. However, if it is believed that the fracture is in an unstable configuration and further loss of fixation may occur, open reduction and internal fixation is recommended. Malunion may result. This is usually well tolerated if the tuberosities are well reduced in relation to the humeral head. Displacement at the surgical neck is well tolerated in comparison with that of the tuberosities.

Superficial infections of the pins have been reported. Jaberg et al. [7] reported seven superficial pin tract infections, which were treated with local debridement and antibiotics. There was one deep infection in a diabetic patient. In his series, the pins were left through the skin. Because of this risk, we prefer to cut the pins deep to the skin.

Conclusion

Percutaneous pinning of proximal humerus fractures requires a thorough three-dimensional understanding of proximal humeral anatomy. Placement of the pins can be difficult and dangerous if the pins exit the bone incorrectly or penetrate nearby neurovascular structures. Assessment of reduction and stability can be challenging. The surgeon must be able to use the two-dimensional image obtained on fluoroscopy to assess a three-dimensional reduction. Success of this procedure is also dependent upon patient selection. Only fractures that can be stably reduced with pins are appropriate for this procedure. The four-part valgus-impacted proximal humerus fracture is generally very stable after reduction and is easily amenable to this type of treatment. Excessive comminution of the proximal shaft, especially the medial calcar area, indicates a fracture that may require open treatment with more secure fixation. The surgeon should always be prepared to convert to an open reduction and internal fixation if percutaneous pinning becomes difficult or impossible. In spite of the above concerns, successful percutaneous pinning in an appropriate patient

offers significant advantages over open treatment in a valgus-impacted four-part proximal humerus fracture. Benefits include less dissection and the ability to take advantage of the intact soft tissue sleeve that exists in these proximal humerus fractures. The procedure is shorter in terms of operative time and results in less blood loss. Additional advantages may include less scar formation and possibly accelerated rehabilitation. As our experience with percutaneous pinning increases and we become more familiar with this technique, we will likely see expanding indications for percutaneous pinning.

References

1. Neer CS II. Displaced proximal humeral fractures. II. Treatment of three-part and four-part displacement. J Bone Joint Surg Am, 1970. **52**(6):1090–1103.
2. Neer CS II. Displaced proximal humeral fractures. I. Classification and evaluation. J Bone Joint Surg Am, 1970. **52**(6):1077–1089.
3. Jakob RP, Kristiansen T, Mayo K, et al. Classification and aspects of treatment of fractures of the proximal humerus. In: Bateman J, Welsh R editors. Surgery of the Shoulder. Philadelphia, PA: B. C. Decker, 1984
4. Probe RA. Minimally invasive fixation of tibial pilon fractures. Oper Tech Orthop, 2001. **11**(3):205–217.
5. Kanlic EM, Pesantez RF, Pachon CM. Minimally invasive plate osteosynthesis of the femur. Oper Tech Orthop, 2001. **11**(3):156–167.
6. Morgan S, Jeray K. Minimally invasive plate osteosynthesis in fractures of the tibia. Oper Tech Orthop, 2001. **11**(3):195–204.
7. Jaberg H, Warner JJP, Jakob RP. Percutaneous stabilization of unstable fractures of the humerus. J Bone Joint Surg Am, 1992. **74A**(4):508–515.
8. Resch H, Povacz P, Frohlich R, et al. Percutaneous fixation of three- and four-part fractures of the proximal humerus. J Bone Joint Surg Br, 1997. **79**(2):295–300.
9. Chen CY, Chao EK, Tu YK, et al. Closed management and percutaneous fixation of unstable proximal humerus fractures. J Trauma, 1998. **45**(6):1039–1045.
10. Bohler J. Perkutane oisteosynthese mit dem Rontyenbildrier-Starker. Wiener Klin Wachenschr, 1962. **74**:485–487.
11. Jakob RP, Miniaci A, Anson PS, et al. Four-part valgus impacted fractures of the proximal humerus. J Bone Joint Surg Br, 1991. **73**(2):295–298.
12. Resch H, Beck E, Bayley I. Reconstruction of the valgus-impacted humeral head fracture. J Shoulder Elbow Surg, 1995. **4**:73–80.

13. deAnquin CE, deAnquin CA. Prosthetic replacement in the treatment of serious fractures of the proximal humerus. In: Bayley I, and Lessel L, editors. Shoulder Surgery, Berlin, Springer. 1982:207–217.

14. Stableforth PG. Four-part fractures of the neck of the humerus. J Bone Joint Surg Br. 1984. 66(1):104–108.

15. Laing PG. The arterial supply of the adult humerus. J Bone Joint Surg Am, 1956. 38A:1105–1116.

16. Gerber C, Schneeberger AG, Vinh TS. The arterial vascularization of the humeral head. An anatomical study. J Bone Joint Surg Am, 1990. 72(10):1486–1494.

17. Wheeler DL, Colville MR. Biomechanical comparison of intramedullary and percutaneous pin fixation for proximal humeral fracture fixation. J Orthop Trauma, 1997. 11(5):363–367.

18. Soete P, Clayson P, Costenoble V. Transitory percutaneous pinning in fractures of the proximal humerus. J Shoulder Elbow Surg, 1999. 8(6):569–573.

19. Rowles DJ, McGrory JE. Percutaneous pinning of the proximal part of the humerus. An anatomic study. J Bone Joint Surg Am, 2001. 83A(11): 1695–1699.

Mini-incision Shoulder Arthroplasty

Sara L. Edwards, Theodore A. Blaine, John-Erik Bell, Chad J. Marion, and Louis U. Bigliani

Minimal disruption of soft tissue and a potential for a faster recovery are very attractive benefits of minimally invasive surgery (MIS). MIS, however, must meet the same standards and offer the same successful outcomes as traditional operations performed through larger skin incisions. While mini-incision hip and knee replacement surgery have become accepted techniques, there are no reports to date on mini-incision shoulder arthroplasty (MISA). The goals of MISA are to decrease trauma to surrounding soft tissues, accelerate postoperative rehabilitation, and decrease operative blood loss and complications. Currently, there are two techniques available to achieve the necessary exposure to perform MISA: (1) a concealed axillary incision or (2) a mini-deltopectoral incision. The use of these techniques is based upon the pathology, the severity of disease, the instrumentation, and the surgeon's experience.

Indications

Glenohumeral Arthritis

Many patients undergoing shoulder arthroplasty for arthritis require extensive releases and exposure to properly address the pathology.

The decision to perform MISA vs. traditional incisions must therefore be made by the surgeon based on each individual patient's pathology, the instrumentation available, and the surgeon's experience. While MISA is becoming more common, patients who have large osteophytes, limited range of motion, or who are large and muscular may require a traditional approach. As in all cases of shoulder arthroplasty, preoperative radiographs that include a true anteroposterior (AP) and axillary view are essential for preoperative planning and in deciding whether MISA is a reasonable approach (Figs. 7.1 and 7.2). An axillary radiograph is especially important and a CT scan may also be required to adequately evaluate the glenoid vault. If there is excessive posterior glenoid bone erosion, then a MISA approach is not advisable, because exposure is more difficult. The ideal patient is a thin female with satisfactory range of motion (forward flexion of 100°, external rotation of 20°, and internal rotation to L3) and small osteophytes. Decreased soft tissue disruption and limited detachment of the subscapularis muscle during this approach are beneficial in terms of restoration of subscapularis function and accelerated rehabilitation postoperatively.

Several reports have documented superior range of motion and better pain relief achieved in patients undergoing total shoulder arthroplasty vs. hemiarthroplasty for osteoarthritis [1–3]. Therefore, the decision to perform a hemiarthroplasty instead of total shoulder replacement (TSR) so that the operation may be done through a MISA approach is not recommended.

L.U. Bigliani (✉)
Department of Orthopaedic Surgery,
New York-Presbyterian Hospital,
Columbia University Medical Center,
New York, NY, USA
e-mail: lubl@columbia.edu

G.R. Scuderi and A.J. Tria (eds.), *Minimally Invasive Surgery in Orthopedics: Upper Extremity Handbook*, DOI 10.1007/978-1-4614-0673-0_7, © Springer Science+Business Media, LLC 2012

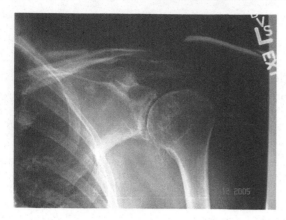

Fig. 7.1 True AP radiograph of a patient with glenohumeral osteoarthritis

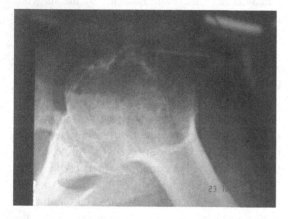

Fig. 7.2 Axillary radiograph of a patient with glenohumeral osteoarthritis

Glenoid pathology in the setting of shoulder arthroplasty usually requires resurfacing with a glenoid component. The decision to perform humeral head replacements (HHR) vs. TSR is based on the pathology and not the approach to be used.

Four-Part Proximal Humerus Fractures

Hemiarthroplasty may be indicated for the treatment of four-part proximal humerus fractures. A minimally invasive approach in HHR for fracture needs to provide adequate exposure for secure tuberosity fixation as well as minimal soft tissue dissection to preserve the biological environment to foster bone healing. New innovative

technological advances in prosthetic design aid the surgeon in achieving these goals. These include a lower profile contour of the proximal stem of the humeral prosthesis so that the tuberosity will fit anatomically. Also, the addition of tantalum, a metal that promotes ingrowth of bone, will allow bone to heal to metal as well as bone. Generally, once the hematoma has been evacuated, the rotator cuff in proximal humerus fractures is healthy and has excellent excursion, obviating the need for extensive surgical releases. We have developed a small jig system that attaches to the prosthesis and allows the surgeon to accurately determine the retroversion and height of the humeral component. Lack of contractures combined with new technology for placement of the prosthesis and fixation of the tuberosities makes the minimally invasive approach an excellent option for these patients.

Avascular Necrosis

While total shoulder arthroplasty has had superior results to hemiarthroplasty in patients with glenohumeral arthritis in several recent series, there are some cases where hemiarthroplasty is the procedure of choice. These include avascular necrosis (Cruess stages I-III, and sometimes IV) where the humeral head is still somewhat concentric and the glenoid is not arthritic. MISA is particularly useful in these patients, since glenoid exposure is not required.

Surgical Technique

Positioning of the arm in space to allow adequate visualization and instrumentation is critically important in all shoulder surgery, and especially in MISA. The beach chair position is used with a modified short arm board on the operative side. The arm board is placed on the distal aspect of the humerus, so the proximal humerus remains free. This allows extension of the arm for humeral shaft preparation as well as a more distal support to hold the arm in a more neutral position. Another option is the hydraulic arm positioner (SPIDER, TENET Medical Engineering, Inc.,

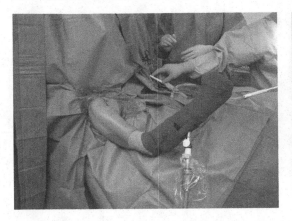

Fig. 7.3 Hydraulic arm positioner used to position the arm in space during MISA

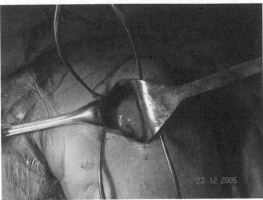

Fig. 7.5 The deltopectoral interval is entered, as per the usual deltopectoral approach

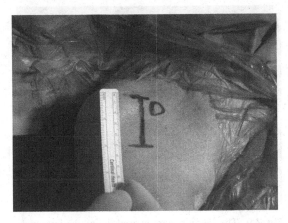

Fig. 7.4 Location of the MISA skin incision, measuring 5 cm (2 in.) just lateral to the coracoid process

Calgary, Alberta, Canada), which eliminates the need for another assistant and also avoids inevitable assistant fatigue in holding the arm throughout the procedure (Fig. 7.3). Rotation of the humerus into both internal and external rotation is essential at different times during the procedure.

Based on cadaveric studies and clinical experience, the authors have found that the current instrumentation used for shoulder arthroplasty tends to exit the skin in a 2-in. (5-cm) arc centered and just lateral to the coracoid process (Fig. 7.4). Furthermore, we and others have also found that the average diameter of the humeral head at the surgical neck is approximately 49 mm [4, 5]. Based on these findings, we think that the skin incision for shoulder arthroplasty must be at least 5 cm (2 in.) to allow placement of a humeral

head component in shoulder arthroplasty, but does not necessarily need to be any larger. The authors have therefore devised a skin incision that is centered just lateral to the coracoid process. This incision can be utilized in MISA for variety of diagnosis. The location of the incision allows better access to the tuberosities in fracture cases and provides adequate glenoid exposure in arthritic disorders. The incision measures approximately 2 in., just enough to deliver the humeral head from the wound. The placement of the starting incision is crucial for this approach. It has to be superior enough to provide direct access to the humeral canal for humeral preparation and placement of the prosthesis as well as allow adequate exposure of the glenoid. Alternatively, the concealed axillary incision is made within the axillary crease skin folds and begins at a point midway between the top of the coracoid and the inferior border of the pectoralis major.

The deltopectoral interval is identified and incised in a similar manner to the traditional anterior approach (Fig. 7.5). Subcutaneous dissection is necessary along the deltopectoral interval superiorly and inferiorly for adequate exposure. Care is taken to protect the attachment of the deltoid to the clavicle and acromion. The cephalic vein is generally retracted with the deltoid muscle secondary to the fact that there are more contributories superiorly from the deltoid than inferiorly from the pectoralis. The pectoralis major is retracted medially, and the deltoid with the cephalic vein is retracted laterally. The deltopectoral interval is developed

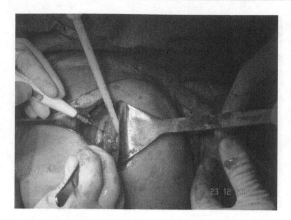

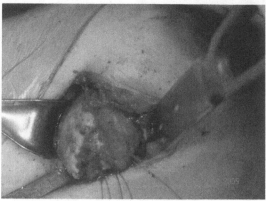

Fig. 7.6 The subscapularis is incised at its insertion to the lesser tuberosity and tagged for later repair

Fig. 7.8 The humeral head is delivered from the wound after releasing the subscapularis tendon insertion

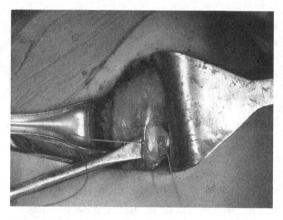

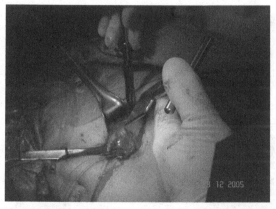

Fig. 7.7 The biceps tendon is located within its groove and tenotomized or tenodesed in the MISA approach

Fig. 7.9 The starter reamer is used to find the intramedullary canal of the humerus

and entered in a similar fashion. After exposure to the subscapularis muscle is achieved, the muscle is detached directly off the lesser tuberosity, superiorly, starting at the rotator interval (Fig. 7.6). The tendon is incised just medial to the biceps tendon, leaving a 2- to 4-mm cuff of tissue for later repair. The rotator interval is also released all the way to the base of the coracoid. In a traditional, more generous incision, the role of biceps tenotomy is debated. MISA, in most cases, requires biceps tenotomy with or without later tenodesis to provide adequate visualization (Fig. 7.7). The subscapularis is detached just enough to deliver the humeral head from the wound (Fig. 7.8). Inferiorly, the subscapularis insertion may be preserved. However, if there is inferior osteophyte formation, then the inferior subscapularis insertion must be detached. The preparation of the humerus is

performed with tapered reamers, which, with an incision based lateral to the coracoid, easily exit the skin (Fig. 7.9). An intramedullary cutting guide is used to make the humeral neck cut. In MISA, this cutting guide must be low profile and should have the ability to be positioned outside the skin incision if necessary (Figs. 7.10 and 7.11). Humeral trials are then performed. Correct alignment of the component is crucial and one has to have adequate visualization; the incision should be enlarged if the visualization is poor. Before placement of the final humeral prosthesis, bone tunnels are made and sutures are passed for future subscapularis repair. If TSR is performed, attention is directed to the glenoid exposure (see following discussion).

Once the glenoid component has been replaced or if hemiarthroplasty alone is performed, humeral trials are placed to determine appropriate sizing

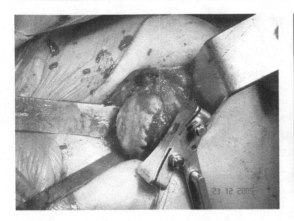

Fig. 7.10 The humeral cutting block is pinned to the humeral neck but is positioned outside the skin

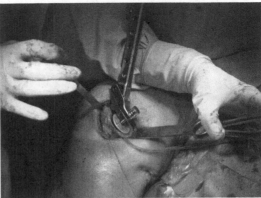

Fig. 7.12 The trial humeral prosthesis is inserted in the appropriate version, as referenced off the humeral insertor

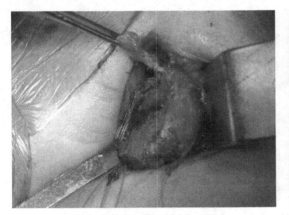

Fig. 7.11 The humeral neck cut has been made, and the humeral head removed

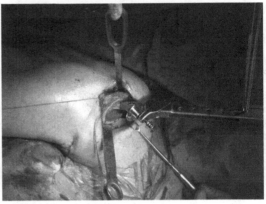

Fig. 7.13 Version rods on the humeral insertor are used to position the prosthesis in the correct version

(Fig. 7.12); it is critical to place the humeral component in the appropriate version (usually 30° retroversion). Shoulder arthroplasty systems that allow version to be determined outside of the wound on the humeral insertors are critical for this step of the MISA procedure (Fig. 7.13). Sutures are now placed in the humeral neck for later repair of the subscapularis as per the surgeon preference.

With the advent of new humeral prostheses that promote proximal bony ingrowth, uncemented humeral components are favored, particularly with the MISA technique (Fig. 7.14). If cementation of the humeral component is performed, a cement restrictor is placed in the humeral canal 2 cm distal to the tip of the prosthesis. Minimal cement is typically concentrated around the metaphyseal

portion of the prosthesis, since it is primarily used to control humeral component rotation.

Once the humeral component is fixed, trial head sizes are performed to reproduce the normal anatomy of the humeral head (Fig. 7.15). This typically requires an offset humeral head component with the maximal offset in the posterosuperior location. Trial reduction is then performed. An appropriate head size will allow translation of the humeral head on the glenoid of approximately 50% of the glenoid surface in any direction. It is very important to avoid overstuffing the glenohumeral joint, which can lead to persistent pain and postoperative stiffness. Once the appropriate head size is determined, the neck is dried with a clean sponge and the final humeral head is impacted on the Morse taper (Fig. 7.16).

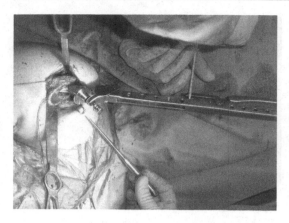

Fig. 7.14 A proximal trabecular metal prosthesis promotes bony ingrowth in the metaphysic

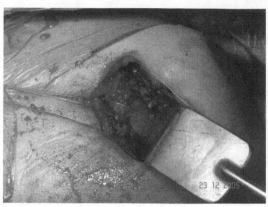

Fig. 7.17 A Fukuda retractor is placed on the posterior rim of the glenoid to allow glenoid visualization

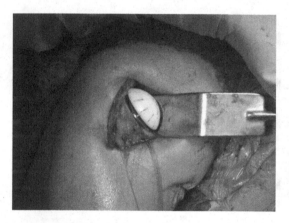

Fig. 7.15 Humeral heads are tested to determine appropriate size and offset

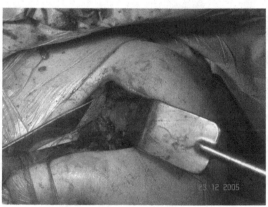

Fig. 7.18 A spiked Darrach retractor is placed on the anterior rim of the glenoid to complete glenoid visualization

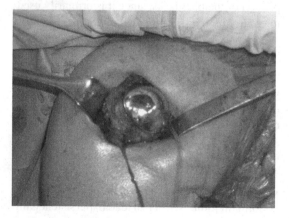

Fig. 7.16 The humeral head component of the prosthesis is impacted on the Morse taper humeral stem

Glenoid Replacement in Total Shoulder Arthroplasty

Glenoid exposure can be challenging even through the traditional incision; therefore, careful patient selection for a minimally invasive approach for total shoulder arthroplasty is required. Proper preparation of the glenoid and placement of the component is crucial. After proper humeral preparation as described previously, a Fukuda or malleable retractor is placed to assess the glenoid (Fig. 7.17). This helps retract the humerus laterally and posteriorly. An anterior spiked narrow Darrach retractor (Fig. 7.18) is then placed on the anterior rim of the glenoid. The provisional humeral stem is left in the canal during glenoid exposure and preparation. This helps to protect the integrity of the humeral stem during retraction.

To achieve adequate exposure to the glenoid, capsular release superiorly, anteriorly, and inferiorly around the glenoid is performed. Care is taken to protect the axillary nerve by staying directly on the humeral neck inferiorly and retracting the inferior capsule in an inferior direction with a Darrach retractor. For routine total shoulder arthroplasty where instability is not a problem and the rotator cuff is usually intact, an anterior capsulectomy may be performed to improve exposure. This should not proceed below the 6 o'clock position (inferior glenoid) to avoid injury to the axillary nerve. A special spiked Darrach retractor is placed anteriorly for adequate visualization. In thin patients with good range of motion and minimal glenoid deformity, this is usually enough for adequate visualization and reaming of the glenoid. Reaming is performed to achieve concentric stable fit of the glenoid component in appropriate version. Pegged or keeled glenoid components may be used. In one study, pegged glenoids were found to have superior fixation to keeled glenoids as well as decreased lucent lines, so we prefer to use pegged glenoid components. Dual-radius glenoid design can also be implemented to use smaller instruments to match a larger head size. The dual-radius implant has a small-radius base with a larger-radius articular surface, allowing easier implantation of the glenoid. Cement is pressurized in the pegged or keeled vault (Fig. 7.19).

Soft Tissue Repair and Wound Closure

Once the glenoid component is placed, attention is turned back to the humerus. The trial humeral stem is removed. A 2-mm hand-held drill is used to make three drill holes. The first hole is made

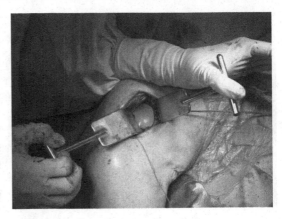

Fig. 7.19 The final glenoid component is placed through the mini-incision

on the superior aspect of the lesser tuberosity from outside to inside the humeral shaft. A #2 nonabsorbable braided suture is passed with a free needle first through the lateral cuff of tendon and then through the drill hole, from outside to in, and tagged with a free clamp. Two parallel holes are drilled across the superior half of the lesser tuberosity, in a medial to lateral direction, spaced approximately 1 cm apart. Often it is necessary to drill the tunnel from both the medial and lateral side, angling slightly to allow the two sides to meet. Two #2 nonabsorbable sutures are placed in a medial to lateral direction through the tunnels. These are tagged for later use. The humeral component and the humeral head are placed as described above.

After placement of the humeral component, the arm should be placed in 20–30° of external rotation. A marking suture can be placed in the superior aspect of the tendon to set the tension for the rest of the repair. Working superiorly to inferiorly, the superior bone tunnel suture is used. This sequence is repeated with the other two bone tunnel sutures, bringing the medial edge of the suture under the corresponding tissue of subscapularis. Interrupted simple sutures are placed in the remaining superior tendon, and can be placed in between the bone tunnel sutures for added protection. More inferiorly, figure-of-eight sutures are

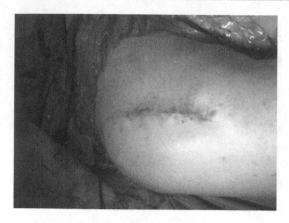

Fig. 7.20 The MISA incision is closed with an absorbable running monofilament subcuticular suture with tails left out of the wound

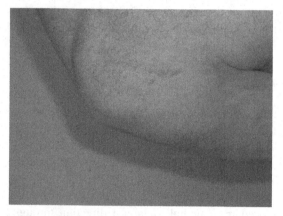

Fig. 7.21 Final appearance of the MISA incision when healed (1 year postoperatively)

placed. This portion of the procedure is critically important because subscapularis failure is the most common early complication of shoulder arthroplasty. Overtensioning must be avoided, because this can lead to necrosis and rupture. The rotator interval is left open to prevent stiffness in external rotation. Closure of the wound is performed in the usual fashion, with a running absorbable monofilament suture used to close the skin (Fig. 7.20). Suture tails are left out of the wound and secured with Steri-strips; these are clipped in the office at the 2-week follow-up visit. Intraoperative AP radiographs are taken in all cases to verify the size and position of the prosthesis before leaving the operating room.

Postoperative Care

Postoperative care is a critical component of managing patients after minimally invasive shoulder arthroplasty. Because of decreased soft tissue damage, patients tend to have a faster recovery time. Despite the patient's eagerness to get back to functional activities, the standard postoperative rehabilitation program must be followed at this early stage of implementation of this technique. The amount of time that is required for soft tissue healing is still the same regardless of the approach.

Results

We reviewed the results of the first 12 consecutive patients with shoulder arthroplasty performed through a mini-incision by two shoulder arthroplasty surgeons. Diagnoses included osteoarthritis (6 cases), fracture (2 cases), avascular necrosis (3 cases), and cuff tear arthropathy (1 case). There were six HHR and six TSR. One of two mini-incisions was used: (1) a 5- to 6-cm incision just lateral to the coracoid process, or (2) a 7- to 8-cm concealed axillary incision below the coracoid process. The average incision length was 6.2 cm (range 5–8 cm). A biceps tenotomy with tenodesis was performed in all patients where the biceps was present at surgery.

At the 6-month (on average) follow-up (range, 65–445 days), no patient reported significant pain postoperatively, and all but the one patient with cuff tear arthropathy had a successful result. There were two transient complications (temporary musculocutaneous nerve palsy and postoperative wound drainage), both of which resolved without incident. The musculocutaneous nerve palsy is thought to be related to excessive retraction required in the more medially based axillary incision; this incision has more recently been abandoned in favor of the incision lateral to the coracoid described in this article. Since using this incision, we have noted a high level of patient satisfaction, and the final cosmesis from this incision has been favored by our patients (Fig. 7.21).

Conclusions

Minimally invasive approaches for shoulder arthroplasty may offer improved patient cosmesis, faster recovery, and less soft tissue trauma. As these techniques continue to develop and patient demand increases, the development of new instrumentation (retractors, cutting guides, component insertion/removal instruments) may make MISA the preferred technique for many shoulder surgeons. Early results using currently available instruments and techniques have been encouraging and support the further advancement of minimally invasive approaches to shoulder arthroplasty.

References

1. Jain NB, Hocker S, Pietrobon R, et al. Total arthroplasty versus hemiarthroplasty for glenohumeral osteoarthritis: role of provider volume. J Shoulder Elbow Surg. 2005 Jul–Aug;14(4):361–7.
2. Rickert M, Loew M. Hemiarthroplasty or total shoulder replacement in glenohumeral osteoarthritis? Orthopade. 2007 Nov;36(11):1013–6.
3. Haines JF, Trail IA, Nuttall D, Birch A, Barrow A. The results of arthroplasty in osteoarthritis of the shoulder. J Bone Joint Surg Br. 2006 Apr;88(4):496–501.
4. Blaine TA, et al. American Shoulder and Elbow Surgeons Focus Conference, November 13–16, 2003.
5. Iannotti JP, Spencer EE, Winter U, Deffenbaugh D, Williams G. Prosthetic positioning in total shoulder arthroplasty. J Shoulder Elbow Surg. 2005 Jan-Feb; 14(1 Suppl S):111S–121S.

Overview of Elbow Approaches: Small Incisions or Arthroscopic Portals

8

Bradford O. Parsons

Surgical management of patients with elbow pathology has evolved substantially in recent years. Technical improvements in fracture care, arthritis, and other pathologic conditions have led to more predictable restoration of function and relief of pain in many patients. Along with advances in elbow surgery has come the idea of "minimally invasive" surgery in orthopedics. Patients often ask for the mini-incision hip or knee surgery, and the elbow is no different. Minimally invasive techniques potentially allow for less perioperative pain, less morbidity, and faster recovery in properly selected patients. The literature is rife with reports describing less invasive surgical techniques for managing elbow conditions, especially arthroscopic techniques [1–20]. Although this "wave of enthusiasm" has led to a shift from traditional open techniques to arthroscopic surgery in many elbow conditions, the principles of surgical management must remain the same, i.e., the pathologic lesions must be appropriately addressed. This chapter serves as an overview of how we can transition from traditional open techniques to minimally invasive or arthroscopic techniques for many elbow problems.

Elbow Surgical Anatomy

The elbow is a complex joint whose main function is to enable positioning the hand in space. Morrey has described the functional range of motion of the elbow to be from 30° to 130° in flexion–extension and a 100° arc of supination and pronation (evenly divided) [21]. Often patients will lose motion after trauma, and stiffness is the rule, not the exception in many situations. Stiffness can be a result of intrinsic and extrinsic contractures as well as heterotopic bone, resulting in distorted anatomy. As with any orthopedic procedure, it is critical to understand the three-dimensional anatomy and anatomical relationships of the elbow prior to performing surgery, especially when performing minimally invasive or arthroscopic techniques, where surgical exposure is potentially limited. It is beyond the scope of this text to review all of the anatomy of the elbow, but a few principles should be discussed, specifically the location of the nerves and ligaments around the elbow.

The relationship of the neurovascular structures to the elbow is critical when attempting minimally invasive or arthroscopic elbow procedures. Portal placement around the elbow for arthroscopy is mainly based on the relationship of these structures to the osseous anatomy. The most frequently encountered nerve during elbow surgery is the ulnar nerve. The ulnar nerve lies in the cubital tunnel posterior to the medial epicondyle and therefore medial-sided procedures such as cubital tunnel release, medial column contracture

B.O. Parsons (✉)
Department of Orthopaedics, Mount Sinai School of Medicine, New York, NY, USA
e-mail: bradford.parsons@mountsinai.org

G.R. Scuderi and A.J. Tria (eds.), *Minimally Invasive Surgery in Orthopedics: Upper Extremity Handbook*,
DOI 10.1007/978-1-4614-0673-0_8, © Springer Science+Business Media, LLC 2012

release, or medial column fractures require identification of the ulnar nerve. Transposition of the nerve following trauma or other conditions may be necessary but often cannot be performed via a mini-incision.

The radial nerve is also frequently encountered, especially the posterior interosseous branch. The radial nerve usually bifurcates into superficial and posterior interosseous branches at the leading edge of the supinator. Lateral-based procedures such as two-incision biceps repair, radial head fractures, or lateral column procedures require an understanding of the location of the radial nerve. The median nerve lies medial to the bicipital aponeurosis and brachial artery. It may be encountered during medial-sided or anterior elbow approaches, such as single-incision biceps repairs, contracture release, or coronoid fractures.

The ligamentous anatomy is critical to the stability of the elbow, with the medial collateral ligament (MCL) and the lateral ulnar collateral ligament (LUCL) acting as primary stabilizers of the elbow. Violation of these ligaments iatrogenically can result in elbow instability. The MCL originates off of the anterior face of the medial epicondyle and inserts on the ulna at the sublime tubercle. It lies deep to the wrist flexor origin and is confluent with the joint capsule. The LUCL originates from an isometric point on the lateral aspect of the capitellum and courses around the posterolateral aspect of the radial head to insert on the supinator crest of the ulna. It is also confluent with the capsule laterally and may be encountered during lateral approaches to the elbow. Regardless of the surgical approach around the elbow, the close proximity of these important structures requires a thorough understanding of their anatomy.

When to Attempt a Minimally Invasive Elbow Procedure

Although very attractive to patients and surgeons, minimally invasive approaches and procedures are often more technically challenging then their traditional open counterparts. Therefore, it is prudent to perform these minimally invasive techniques only with thorough understanding of the three-dimensional anatomy of the elbow. Additionally,

a surgeon should be comfortable and competent with the principles of the traditional open techniques, as the pathology has not changed, and therefore the surgical principles must remain the same. The patient must be an appropriate candidate as well. Patients with distorted anatomy, such as end-stage rheumatoid arthritis or posttraumatic arthritis, previous surgery with scarring, or complex fractures, are often not amenable to minimally invasive techniques. Patients who are very muscular or obese also may not be candidates for minimally invasive open procedures, but arthroscopy is usually not precluded by these factors.

Pathologic entities that are amenable to minimally invasive open techniques include tennis elbow release, medial epicondylitis, collateral ligament reconstruction, biceps or triceps tendon repair, and isolated radial head, capitellar, or olecranon fractures. Advances in elbow arthroscopic technique and instrumentation have enabled many surgeons to "push the envelope" of what can safely and effectively be addressed with arthroscopy. Originally used mainly for removal of loose bodies [7], arthroscopy has been successfully used for treatment of tennis elbow, posttraumatic contracture release, synovectomy, osteocapsular arthroplasty, osteochondral lesions, capitellar and coronoid fractures, and pediatric elbow conditions [1–4, 7, 8, 11–14, 19, 20]. Although these advances have enabled experienced elbow arthroscopists and surgeons to manage increasingly complex conditions, many conditions are often not amenable to minimally invasive or arthroscopic techniques. This includes complex distal humerus or elbow fracture–dislocations, total elbow arthroplasty, complex contractures with heterotopic bone (although these can be occasionally addressed with arthroscopy in experienced hands), and revision procedures, especially when there is distorted osseous or neurovascular anatomy.

Minimally Invasive Open Approaches

As stated above, certain elbow conditions are amenable to minimally invasive open approaches. Extensile approaches to the elbow include the medial and lateral column approaches [22] and

Fig. 8.1 Skin incision for the standard Kocher approach. A curvilinear incision is made over the lateral epicondyle and lateral column proximally, extending distally across the radial head

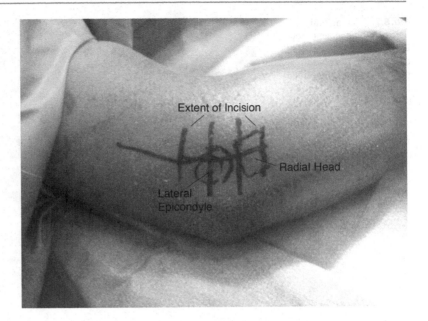

the posterior approach [23, 24]. These approaches, or some variation of them, are the "workhorse" approaches to the elbow and allow excellent exposure and versatility to manage many conditions. However, they are extensile and would not be considered minimally invasive. Other approaches are less extensile and could be considered minimally invasive; these include approaches used for open tennis elbow release, one-incision or two-incision biceps tendon repairs, MCL reconstruction, and some fractures. Many of these specific entities will be discussed in later chapters and therefore we will not address them here. However, one approach is not discussed later and warrants discussion here; that is the Kocher approach to the lateral elbow.

Kocher Approach

Traditionally, the Kocher approach has been used to manage laterally based fractures or ligament injuries, such as radial head or capitellar fractures. This approach can be considered minimally invasive with small incisions in properly selected situations and patients. The Kocher approach utilizes the interval between the anconeus (posteriorly) and the extensor carpi ulnaris (ECU) (laterally). The posterior interosseous nerve (PIN) is

in close proximity during the Kocher approach, and, to protect the PIN, the forearm is maintained in pronation. Although frequently used, two concerns regarding the Kocher approach should be raised. First, the classic Kocher approach is not extensile distally, as the PIN crosses the field distal to the annular ligament. Second, the interval between the ECU and anconeus traverses across the course of the LUCL, and this structure must be protected during this approach. One option is to use the interval between the extensor carpi radialis longus (ECRL) and the extensor digitorum comminus (EDC), a more anterior interval. This interval is in the anterior hemisphere of the capitellum and radial head, where most fractures occur, and will not violate the LUCL. The skin incision is made just slightly anterior then that for the Kocher along the same course.

The patient is positioned supine for the Kocher approach, with the arm on a hand table or over the chest. A tourniquet can be used if desired. The posterior and lateral osseous landmarks of the elbow are marked on the skin, including the lateral epicondyle, lateral column, radial head, and capitellum. The skin incision is marked as a curvilinear incision from just proximal to the lateral epicondyle to the radial head (Fig. 8.1). The skin is incised to the level of the fascia and skin flaps are made.

Fig. 8.2 The interval between the anconeus and ECU (Kocher's interval) can often be identified by a "fat stripe" (identified by the *forceps* and *broad solid line*)

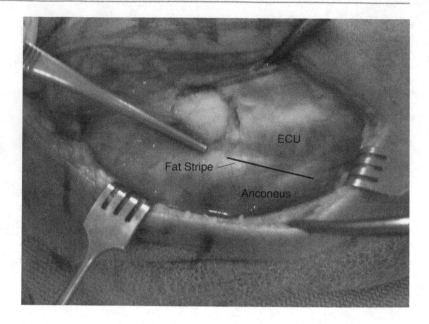

The interval between the ECU and the anconeus is often identifiable by a "fat stripe" and the fascia and muscle are incised in this fat stripe (Fig. 8.2). Careful dissection can then allow for identification of the supinator muscle distally (with fibers oriented transversely vs. longitudinally for the extensors) and the capsule of the joint. Often, in trauma, the capsule is torn laterally, exposing the joint. The LUCL must be identified at this point. It is in the posterior hemisphere of the capitellum, as previously described. If an arthrotomy is necessary, it must be made at the level of the anterior half of the capitellum and radial head so as to not violate the LUCL. The joint and osseous structures of the lateral aspect of the elbow are now exposed via the arthrotomy. The capsule can be further elevated off of the distal humerus anteriorly if needed.

After completion of the procedure, it is critical to repair the capsular arthrotomy anatomically. The muscular interval must also be closed, and heavy nonabsorbable suture should be used. If injury to the LUCL has been encountered, this also must be anatomically repaired, either with anchors or (my preference) bone tunnels at the isometric point. The skin is closed in layers by surgeon preference after hemostasis has been obtained.

Elbow Arthroscopy

Elbow arthroscopy has evolved substantially over recent years. Originally performed for "simple" loose body removal or diagnostic procedures, the arthroscope now is utilized for management of complex arthritis, contractures, and some fractures of the elbow. The ability to perform these more complex procedures has been enabled by improvement in instrumentation and arthroscopic technique, and by thorough understanding of the three-dimensional anatomy of the elbow. This section details the indications and contraindications of elbow arthroscopy as well as positioning, portal placement, and technical tips on avoiding complications.

Indications

Many procedures typically performed "open" are now performed arthroscopically in experienced surgeons' hands. The pathologic entities now treated via arthroscopic techniques include tennis elbow, osteochondral lesions and loose body excision, synovectomy, capsular release, osteocapsular arthroplasty, and some intraarticular fractures

[1–4, 7, 8, 11–14, 19, 20]. When transitioning from open to arthroscopic techniques, the surgeon must have a thorough understanding of the surgical principles of the open procedures. It is suggested that when beginning elbow arthroscopy, one should start with less complex procedures, such as tennis elbow release or loose body removal. As surgeon experience and technical abilities increase, procedures that are more complicated can be performed.

Contraindications

Contraindications to elbow arthroscopy include patients who have significant derangement of the normal osseous and neurovascular anatomy of the elbow [15]. This would include patients who have had previous ulnar nerve transposition, as the transposed nerve lies in the path of the anteromedial portal of the elbow. In these patients, the nerve must be identified prior to medial portal placement. Additionally, patients with substantial posttraumatic or inflammatory arthritic changes with loss of the normal osseous architecture makes appropriate portal placement difficult, placing neurovascular structures at risk. Patients with substantial heterotopic ossification are often contraindicated because of the derangement of the normal neurovascular anatomy. Finally, patients with a history of previous surgery should be carefully considered for arthroscopy, as normal anatomic relationships may have been altered by the previous surgery.

Instrumentation

A standard 4.0-mm, 30°-offset arthroscope is used for elbow arthroscopy. Smaller arthroscopes are typically not necessary. It is preferable to use inflow cannulas without side vents, as the vents may lie outside the capsule and therefore can contribute to fluid extravasation and soft tissue swelling [25]. Standard arthroscopic shavers and burrs can be used, as well as standard arthroscopic graspers and biters. Cannulas help maintain portal positions and should be used routinely, and trochars should be blunt tipped to minimize iatrogenic injury of neurovascular and articular structures. Blunt-tipped switching sticks should also be available to serve as retractors for improved visualization. "Elbow arthroscopy sets" with standard instruments, including cannulated dilators, cannulas, and grasping instruments are now commercially available if desired (Arthrex, Naples, FL).

Patient Positioning

Patients can be positioned in three different manners for elbow arthroscopy, depending upon surgeon preference. We use the lateral decubitus position, with the arm placed over a post and draped free. Alternatively, the prone position can be used, and some prefer the supine position with the arm held in an extremity positioner such as the McConnel arm holder (McConnell Orthopaedics Co., Greenville, TX). Each position has its advantages and disadvantages. We will discuss the lateral position here.

Patients are positioned in lateral decubitus on a beanbag with bony prominences well padded. Care is taken to ensure that the patient is brought to the edge of the operating room table to allow for full exposure of the extremity. The contralateral arm is flexed and placed on an armrest out of the way. A tourniquet is placed on the proximal brachium, and draped out of the field. The operative arm is abducted 90° at the shoulder with the elbow flexed 90° over a post, so that the brachium is parallel to the floor and the elbow is completely free and can be easily flexed and extended without impingement (Fig. 8.3). Care must be taken to use an arm post that will allow for easy instrumentation proximally along the brachium, and that the post is very proximal so that the elbow is completely free.

Arthroscopy Set-Up

Either pump or gravity insufflation may be used for elbow arthroscopy. If a pump is used, the pressure should be kept no higher then 30 mmHg.

Fig. 8.3 Lateral decubitus positioning for elbow arthroscopy. The patient's operative arm is abducted 90° and the elbow is flexed over a padded post, taking care to ensure that access to the arm is not restricted. The forearm should hang free and allow for unrestricted range of motion of the elbow

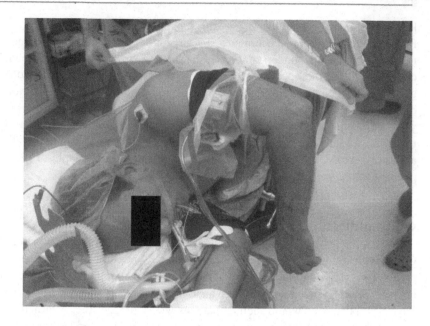

Unlike other joints, the elbow is subcutaneous and very susceptible to swelling of the soft tissues during arthroscopy. Once substantial soft tissue swelling has occurred, the complexity and difficulty of the elbow arthroscopy dramatically increases. Rather then increasing pump pressure to improve visualization, it is preferable to use retractors.

Outflow cannulas can be used and are set to either gravity or pump. If motorized instruments (shavers, burrs) are used, the outflow of these instruments should be set to gravity, not to suction, because exuberant suction can increase the chance that neurovascular structures may be pulled into the instrument and injured.

The osseous landmarks of the elbow are marked, including the lateral epicondyle, the radial head and capitellum, the medial epicondyle, the ulnar nerve, and the olecranon tip. The typical portals are also marked, including the proximal anteromedial, straight posterior (transtriceps), proximal posterolateral, and anterolateral. Accessory portals may be used in addition to the standard portals for retraction, etc. (Figs. 8.4 and 8.5). Each portal is discussed further below.

The joint is insufflated with ~20 mL normal saline via the lateral "soft spot" (the triangular area bounded by the lateral epicondyle, radial head, and olecranon). Realize that, in the contracted joint, insufflation may be more difficult because of the noncompliant capsule [6, 10, 18, 20, 26]. Joint insufflation is valuable in distending the capsule and increasing the distance of the neurovascular structures from the joint, but does not change the distance of these structures from the capsule, and therefore these structures are still in close proximity when performing capsular procedures.

The elbow has two main compartments, anterior and posterior. Even in experienced hands, swelling can be an issue and therefore many surgeons will start in the compartment with greater pathology (i.e., anteriorly for a tennis elbow release, or posteriorly for an arthritic elbow with olecranon osteophytes and extension loss). Preoperative planning should assess which compartment is more pathologic and guide the surgical approach.

Similarly, some variation exists regarding which portals are used to initially visualize the joint. Anteriorly, the two standard options include visualization via the proximal anteromedial portal or via the anterolateral portal. Our standard is to use the proximal anteromedial portal to first visualize the joint, as the literature has shown that this portal is further from neurovascular structures then the lateral portals [1, 27]. We then establish the lateral portal via an outside–in technique with a spinal needle. However, either

Fig. 8.4 Medial sided portals of elbow arthroscopy. The proximal anteromedial portal is approximately 2 cm proximal to the medial epicondyle and anterior to the intermuscular septum. The ulnar nerve should be marked and palpated to ensure that a subluxing nerve is not present

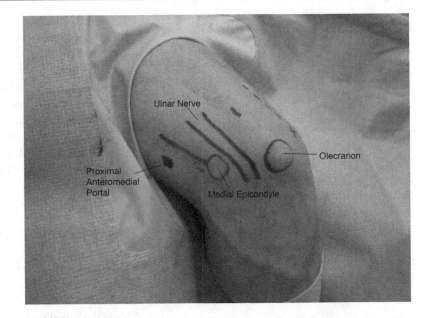

Fig. 8.5 Lateral sides portals of elbow arthroscopy. The proximal anterolateral portal is proximal to the capitellum along the column of the distal humerus. Anterolateral portals more distal (at the level of the radial head) can risk injury to the radial nerve

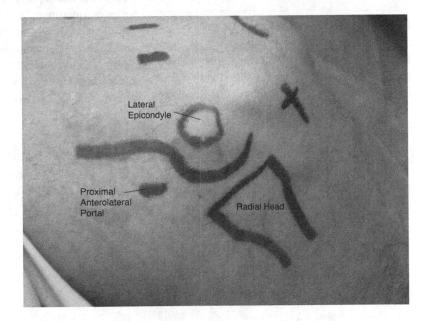

option is viable and many surgeons start with the lateral portal. Posteriorly, most surgeons utilize the transtriceps (posterocentral) portal for initial visualization.

Portal Placement

Many different portals have been utilized for elbow arthroscopy, and the standard portals will be discussed. All portals are placed in an effort to avoid injury to the neurovascular structures around the elbow, but these structures are in close proximity and iatrogenic injury is possible with any of the portals [6, 10, 18, 26, 28–34]. When making portals, only the skin should be incised, and "plunging" of the scalpel should be avoided. Portals are distended with a blunt hemostat or commercially available cannulated dilators.

Proximal Anteromedial Portal

Described by Poehling et al. [35] this portal is located anterior to the intermuscular septum and 2 cm proximal to the medial epicondyle (Fig. 8.4). The ulnar nerve is at greatest risk with this portal, and is typically located 3–4 mm posterior to this portal. After skin incision, the trochar is used to palpate the intermuscular septum and then the portal is established anteriorly. An effort should be made to enter the joint as medial as possible by bringing the trochar base close to the brachium, as this will improve visualization of the anterior compartment. Once the joint is entered, the radial head and capitellum is identified to confirm placement, and then evaluation of the anterior compartment is performed.

Proximal Anterolateral Portal

Described by Field et al. [28] this portal is located 1–2 cm proximal to the lateral epicondyle, just anterior to the humerus (Fig. 8.5). Often this portal is made via an outside-in technique while visualizing from the medial side. The radial nerve is closest to this portal and at highest risk, although it is anterior to the sulcus between the radial head and capitellum. A "safe zone" for lateral portals includes the area bounded by the sulcus between the radial head and capitellum and the proximal anterolateral portal 2 cm proximal [28]. Proximal to the capitellum along the lateral column is safer then distally if accessory portals are needed for retractors, etc.

Transtriceps (Posterocentral) Portal

This portal is made 3 cm proximal to the olecranon process in the midline, which is proximal to the triceps muscle–tendon junction (Fig. 8.6). This is the initial portal when visualizing the posterior compartment, and the majority of the compartment can be visualized, including both medial and lateral gutters and the olecranon articulation. The posterior antebrachial cutaneous nerve and ulnar nerve are at risk with this portal but are both approximately 2 cm away [25].

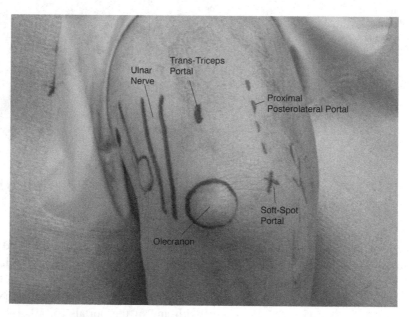

Fig. 8.6 Posterior portals of elbow arthroscopy. The transtriceps (posterocentral) portal is 2 cm proximal to the olecranon tip, in the center of the arm, whereas the accessory proximal posterolateral portal is at the same level but just lateral to the edge of the triceps tendon. Additional accessory portals are possible more distal in line with the accessory proximal posterolateral portal (*dashed lines*). The soft spot portal (marked by an "*x*") is made in the center of the triangle subtended by the radial head, olecranon, and lateral epicondyle

Proximal Posterolateral Portal

Often this is the initial working portal of the posterior compartment. It is made 2–3 cm proximal to the olecranon on the lateral border of the triceps (Fig. 8.6). The trochar is directed toward the olecranon fossa. The posterior and posterolateral gutter structures can be visualized via this portal. The medial and posterior antebrachial cutaneous nerves are at most risk, but are both approximately 2.5 cm away from this portal [29].

"Soft Spot" (Direct Lateral) Portal

This portal is located in the soft spot, the triangular area bounded by the lateral epicondyle, radial head, and olecranon (Fig. 8.6). This portal is often made under direct visualization while viewing from the proximal posterolateral portal, localized with a spinal needle. The posterior antebrachial cutaneous nerve is on average 7 mm from this portal [25]. This portal allows visualization of the posterior capitellum and posterior proximal radioulnar joint. It is often utilized in the management of intraarticular plica or osteochondral lesions of the capitellum.

Tips and Tricks to Avoiding Complications

Avoiding complications centers on avoiding injury to the neurovascular structures around the elbow. The most frequent, and worrisome complication is nerve injury, and injuries to nearly all of the major nerves, or their branches, have been reported [6, 10, 18, 26, 28–34]. The risk of nerve injury has been found to be higher in patients with distorted anatomy, or soft tissue contractures, such as in advanced rheumatoid arthritis or post-traumatic arthropathies [6]. Osseous landmarks should be clearly marked before beginning, as surface landmarks will changes as the elbow swells during arthroscopy. A thorough understanding of the three-dimensional anatomy is critical to avoiding iatrogenic nerve injuries.

Appropriate portal placement decreases the likelihood of nerve injury, as does the use of blunt-tipped trochars. Additionally, keeping the elbow flexed 90° helps relax the anterior capsule and soft tissues, thereby increasing the distance between the joint and neurovascular structures.

Many complications occur as soft tissue swelling distorts anatomy and visualization is compromised. Pump pressure should be kept to a minimum (<30 mmHg) or avoided all together, and intraarticular retractors should be used to increase visualization rather then increasing pump pressure [6]. Suction on motorized shavers and burrs should not be used, as it may draw structures into harm's way. Prior to using elbow arthroscopy, a surgeon should be comfortable with similar open procedures, and, as technical skills are learned, procedures of appropriate complexity should be undertaken. It is suggested that when beginning elbow arthroscopy, one should start with less complex procedures, such as diagnostic procedures, tennis elbow release, or simple loose body excision.

Conclusions

Minimally invasive surgery is a "hot topic" in orthopedics, with many patients desiring the less invasive surgical option. This trend has been observed in nearly all fields of orthopedics, including elbow surgery. Numerous procedures traditionally performed open are now performed via "mini-incisions" or via arthroscopy about the elbow, with good results. This transition has enabled surgeons to treat patients with potentially less morbidity and faster recovery. However, minimally invasive techniques are often more technically demanding then the traditional "open" counterparts, and therefore surgeons should be very comfortable with the standard open procedures prior to attempting less invasive options. With minimally invasive elbow procedures, the key to success is found when patients are appropriately indicated, surgeons have a thorough understanding of the topographical and three-dimensional anatomy, and established techniques are utilized.

References

1. Andrews JR, Carson WG. Arthroscopy of the elbow. Arthroscopy 1985;1(2):97–107.
2. Andrews JR, St Pierre RK, Carson WG, Jr. Arthroscopy of the elbow. Clin Sports Med 1986;5(4):653–62.
3. Baker CL, Brooks AA. Arthroscopy of the elbow. Clin Sports Med 1996;15(2):261–81.
4. Brownlow HC, O'Connor-Read LM, Perko M. Arthroscopic treatment of osteochondritis dissecans of the capitellum. Knee Surg Sports Traumatol Arthrosc 2006;14(2):198–202.
5. Guhl JF. Arthroscopy and arthroscopic surgery of the elbow. Orthopedics 1985;8(10):1290–6.
6. Kelly EW, Morrey BF, O'Driscoll SW. Complications of elbow arthroscopy. J Bone Joint Surg Am 2001;83A(1):25–34.
7. McGinty JB. Arthroscopic removal of loose bodies. Orthop Clin North Am 1982;13(2):313–28.
8. McLaughlin RE, II, Savoie FH, III, Field LD, Ramsey JR. Arthroscopic treatment of the arthritic elbow due to primary radiocapitellar arthritis. Arthroscopy 2006;22(1):63–9.
9. Morrey BF. Arthroscopy of the elbow. Instr Course Lect 1986;35:102–7.
10. Morrey BF. Complications of elbow arthroscopy. Instr Course Lect 2000;49:255–8.
11. Moskal MJ, Savoie FH, III, Field LD. Elbow arthroscopy in trauma and reconstruction. Orthop Clin North Am 1999;30(1):163–77.
12. Mullett H, Sprague M, Brown G, Hausman M. Arthroscopic treatment of lateral epicondylitis: clinical and cadaveric studies. Clin Orthop Relat Res 2005;439:123–8.
13. Noonburg GE, Baker CL, Jr. Elbow arthroscopy. Instr Course Lect 2006;55:87–93.
14. O'Driscoll SW. Elbow arthroscopy for loose bodies. Orthopedics 1992;15(7):855–9.
15. O'Driscoll SW, Morrey BF. Arthroscopy of the elbow. Diagnostic and therapeutic benefits and hazards. J Bone Joint Surg Am 1992;74(1):84–94.
16. Ramsey ML. Elbow arthroscopy: basic setup and treatment of arthritis. Instr Course Lect 2002;51: 69–72.
17. Reddy AS, Kvitne RS, Yocum LA, Elattrache NS, Glousman RE, Jobe FW. Arthroscopy of the elbow: a long-term clinical review. Arthroscopy 2000;16(6): 588–94.
18. Savoie FH, III, Field LD. Arthrofibrosis and complications in arthroscopy of the elbow. Clin Sports Med 2001;20(1):123–9, ix.
19. Savoie FH, III, Nunley PD, Field LD. Arthroscopic management of the arthritic elbow: indications, technique, and results. J Shoulder Elbow Surg 1999;8(3): 214–9.
20. Steinmann SP, King GJ, Savoie FH, III. Arthroscopic treatment of the arthritic elbow. J Bone Joint Surg Am 2005;87(9):2114–21.
21. Morrey BF, Askew LJ, Chao EY. A biomechanical study of normal functional elbow motion. J Bone Joint Surg Am 1981;63(6):872–7.
22. Mansat P, Morrey BF. The column procedure: a limited lateral approach for extrinsic contracture of the elbow. J Bone Joint Surg Am 1998; 80(11):1603–15.
23. Bryan RS, Morrey BF. Extensive posterior exposure of the elbow. A triceps-sparing approach. Clin Orthop Relat Res 1982;(166):88–92.
24. Wadsworth TG. A modified posterolateral approach to the elbow and proximal radioulnar joints. Clin Orthop Relat Res 1979;(144):151–3.
25. Abboud JA, Ricchetti ET, Tjoumakaris F, Ramsey ML. Elbow arthroscopy: basic setup and portal placement. J Am Acad Orthop Surg 2006; 14(5):312–8.
26. Adams JE, Steinmann SP. Nerve injuries about the elbow. J Hand Surg [Am] 2006;31(2):303–13.
27. Lindenfeld TN. Medial approach in elbow arthroscopy. Am J Sports Med 1990;18(4):413–7.
28. Field LD, Altchek DW, Warren RF, O'Brien SJ, Skyhar MJ, Wickiewicz TL. Arthroscopic anatomy of the lateral elbow: a comparison of three portals. Arthroscopy 1994;10(6):602–7.
29. Lynch GJ, Meyers JF, Whipple TL, Caspari RB. Neurovascular anatomy and elbow arthroscopy: inherent risks. Arthroscopy 1986;2(3):190–7.
30. Miller CD, Jobe CM, Wright MH. Neuroanatomy in elbow arthroscopy. J Shoulder Elbow Surg 1995;4(3):168–74.
31. Papilion JD, Neff RS, Shall LM. Compression neuropathy of the radial nerve as a complication of elbow arthroscopy: a case report and review of the literature. Arthroscopy 1988;4(4):284–6.
32. Ruch DS, Poehling GG. Anterior interosseus nerve injury following elbow arthroscopy. Arthroscopy 1997;13(6):756–8.
33. Stothers K, Day B, Regan WR. Arthroscopy of the elbow: anatomy, portal sites, and a description of the proximal lateral portal. Arthroscopy 1995;11(4): 449–57.
34. Thomas MA, Fast A, Shapiro D. Radial nerve damage as a complication of elbow arthroscopy. Clin Orthop Relat Res 1987(215):130–1.
35. Poehling GG, Whipple TL, Sisco L, Goldman B. Elbow arthroscopy: a new technique. Arthroscopy 1989;5(3):222–4.

Mini-incision Medial Collateral Ligament Reconstruction of the Elbow

9

Christopher C. Dodson, Steven J. Thornton, and David W. Altchek

The anterior bundle of the medial collateral ligament (MCL) of the elbow is the primary restraint to valgus load. It has been well documented that throwing athletes are prone to injury of this structure secondary to the repetitive valgus loads subjected to the elbow with overhead pitching [1–4]. Originally described in javelin throwers [5], this injury is almost exclusively seen in overhead-throwing athletes, with baseball pitchers being the most prevalent group of patients. Injury to the MCL has also been shown in wrestlers, tennis players, professional football players, and arm wrestlers [1, 5–7]. Symptomatic valgus instability can arise in these athletes after a MCL injury, thus necessitating operative intervention. Although injury to the MCL in the nonthrowing athlete can have excellent results with nonoperative intervention [8, 9], the overhead throwing athlete may find an injury to the MCL of the elbow to be a career-ending event if surgical intervention is not employed.

Biomechanics and Anatomy

The MCL complex is composed of an anterior bundle, a posterior bundle, and a transverse bundle [10] (Fig. 9.1). The anterior bundle has been

D.W. Altchek (✉)
Department of Orthopaedic Surgery, Weill Medical College of Cornell University, New York, NY, USA

Hospital for Special Surgery, New York, NY, USA
e-mail: altchekd@hss.edu

shown to be the primary restraint to valgus stress at the elbow [11–15]. Injury to the anterior bundle can cause instability of the elbow with subsequent disabling pain in overhead-throwing athletes [9, 16–19]. The humeral origin of both the anterior and posterior bundles is the medial epicondyle. The anterior bundle originates from the anteroinferior aspect of the medial epicondyle [10, 20–22] and inserts at the sublime tubercle of the ulna [10, 22, 23]. On average, the anterior bundle occupies two thirds of the width of the medial epicondyle in the coronal plane [22]. It averages 4.7 mm in width and 27 mm in length [21]. The posterior bundle is triangular, smaller, and fanlike in nature; it originates from the posteroinferior aspect of the medial epicondyle and attaches to the medial olecranon margin [14].

The anterior bundle has separate bands that function as a cam, tightening in a reciprocal fashion as the elbow is flexed and extended [14, 21, 24]. In a cadaveric study, Callaway et al [10]. performed sequential cutting of the MCL while a valgus torque was applied. The anterior band of the anterior bundle was the primary restraint to valgus rotation at 30, 60, and 90° of flexion. The posterior band of the anterior bundle was a coprimary restraint with the anterior band at 120°. In a separate study, Field and Altchek [25] evaluated the laxity seen with MCL injury when viewed through the arthroscope. They found that ulnohumeral joint opening was not visualized in any specimen until complete sectioning of the anterior bundle was performed. However, only 1–2 mm of joint opening was present with complete transaction of the anterior bundle,

G.R. Scuderi and A.J. Tria (eds.), *Minimally Invasive Surgery in Orthopedics: Upper Extremity Handbook*, DOI 10.1007/978-1-4614-0673-0_9, © Springer Science+Business Media, LLC 2012

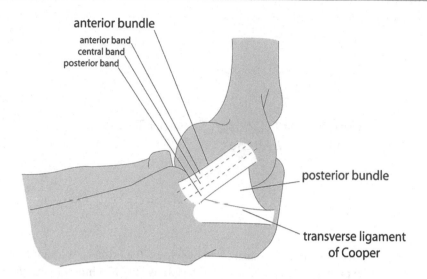

Fig. 9.1 Schematic drawing of the MCL complex. Note that the anterior bundle is composed of three bands. The anterior band of the anterior bundle is the primary restraint to valgus stress (From Dodson CC, Altchek DW. The

Management of Medial Collateral Ligament Tears in the Athlete. Oper Tech Sports Med: 14(2):75–80, 2006, with permission)

emphasizing the subtle exam findings in these athletes. It was shown that the maximum amount of valgus laxity was seen best at 60–75° of flexion.

The flexor carpi ulnaris (FCU) is the predominant muscle overlying the MCL [26]. It is the most posterior structure of the flexor–pronator mass, which places it directly overlying the anterior bundle of the MCL. Thus, the FCU is optimally positioned to provide direct support to the MCL in regards to valgus stability. Preservation of the FCU is important during reconstruction of the MCL in order to maintain one of the secondary restraints to valgus stress. This is further discussed when the surgical technique we currently use is described.

The ulnar nerve lies in close proximity to the MCL. It courses from a point posterior to the medial intermuscular septum above the medial epicondyle toward the anterior aspect of the medial elbow. Once it passes anterior to the intermuscular septum, the ulnar nerve then courses posterior to the medial epicondyle within the cubital tunnel. It then progresses distally to a point just posterior to the sublime tubercle. At this point, the ulnar nerve dives into the FCU, which it innervates. It is important to be familiar with the anatomy of this vulnerable structure

during MCL reconstruction in order to avoid an iatrogenic injury.

History and Physical Examination

In the evaluation of overhead athletes with medial-sided elbow complaints, it is important to first obtain a detailed history. Questions should be posed as to the chronicity of the symptoms as well as its effect on overhead activity. Issues regarding velocity, accuracy, and stamina are important to the throwing athlete and should, therefore, be addressed. It is important to note that many of these athletes will modify their pitching techniques to compensate for the pain; however, these athletes will not be able to reach their maximal throwing velocity secondary to the altered mechanics being implemented. The phase of throwing in which the pain occurs is another important aspect. Conway et al. have shown that nearly 85% of athletes with medial elbow instability will complain of discomfort during the acceleration phase of throwing, in contrast to less than 25% of athletes that will experience pain during the deceleration phase [1]. This same study also showed that up to 40% of patients with MCL injuries may also suffer from ulnar neuritis; [1] therefore, a history of ulnar nerve symptoms should be ascertained as well as information pertaining to the position in which these symptoms are most prevalent.

Patients will present either with an acute event or with an acute on chronic episode. In an acute event, the patient reports having heard a "pop," and subsequently experienced acute medial pain with the inability to continue pitching. In an acute on chronic event, the patient will have experienced an innocuous onset of medial-sided elbow pain over an extended period of time with overhead throwing. This would preclude the acute event as described previously with an inability to continue with full-velocity pitching.

Both passive and active range of motion of the elbow should be documented. During the range of motion testing, attention should be turned to the detection of any crepitus, pain, or mechanical blocks. Patients with valgus overload will frequently develop posteromedial osteophytes that will present as a bony block to full extension. A possible loose body may also present with a similar exam.

Direct palpation of the origin of the MCL is unreliable secondary to the overlying flexor–pronator mass. However, an attempt should be made to elicit discomfort in this region with palpation. The ulnar nerve should be palpated (e.g., Tinel's) to assess for ulnar neuritis or subluxation of the nerve resulting in paresthesias. The medial epicondylar insertion of the flexor pronator mass should also be palpated for tenderness. If the flexor pronator tendon is involved, pain will be reproduced with resisted forearm pronation. This resisted maneuver can help distinguish a MCL injury from a flexor pronator tendonitis.

Several tests to test the MCL have been described. Generally speaking, we typically find the valgus stress test and the moving valgus stress test to be the most specific. To perform the valgus stress test, the examiner places the player's distal forearm under their axilla and applies a valgus load to the elbow in 30° of flexion while palpating the MCL (Fig. 9.2). If the patient complains of increased medial-sided elbow pain or if valgus instability is present, then the test is considered

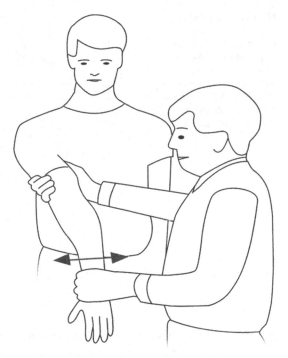

Fig. 9.2 Valgus stress test. While one hand of the examiner supports the elbow, valgus stress is applied with the elbow in approximately 30° of flexion. Tenderness to palpation over the MCL as well as valgus laxity are assessed

positive. However, it must be noted that the amount of instability present in these cases is sometimes too small to be picked up by this maneuver. Therefore, pain may be the only indication of a MCL injury with this test. The moving valgus stress test was originally described by O'Driscoll [27]. This test is performed by applying a valgus stress to the elbow in the flexed position and then quickly extending the elbow. (Fig. 9.3) A positive test produces medial pain typically between 120° and 70° of flexion as a result of shear stress on the MCL. Finally, we also sometimes use the "milking maneuver," which is performed by pulling on the patients thumb with the forearm supinated, the shoulder extended, and the elbow flexed to 90°. A feeling of instability and apprehension along with pain is a positive finding and indicates insufficiency of the posterior band of the anterior bundle.

Posterior impingement secondary to posteromedial olecranon osteophytes should also be assessed. This is accomplished through the valgus

Fig. 9.3 The moving valgus stress test is performed by applying a valgus stress to the maximally flexed elbow and then quickly extending the elbow. A positive test usually produces pain between 120° and 70° of flexion

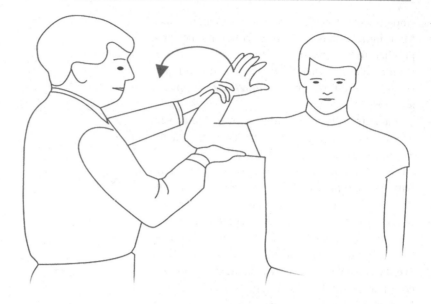

extension overload test. The examiner uses one hand to apply a valgus force across the elbow while stabilizing the elbow joint with the opposite hand. The forearm is placed in a pronated position and the elbow is then quickly brought to full extension while the valgus load is applied. A positive test is indicated by pain in the posteromedial aspect of the elbow.

Imaging

Plain radiographs remain the gold standard for initial evaluation of the elbow. Routine antero-posterior (AP), lateral, and oblique views should be obtained. These standard radiographic views may reveal calcifications in the MCL, medial spurs on the humerus and ulna at the joint line, spurs on the posterior olecranon tip, or loose bodies present in the olecranon fossa (Fig. 9.4). Stress radiographs have been advocated to aid in the diagnosis of MCL tears [28, 29], but we do not routinely use them.

We recommend getting a magnetic resonance imaging (MRI) scan on every patient with a suspected MCL tear. Some studies have shown that the sensitivity of MRI in detecting partial MCL tears is increased by injecting the elbow joint with saline prior to imaging [30]. At the Hospital

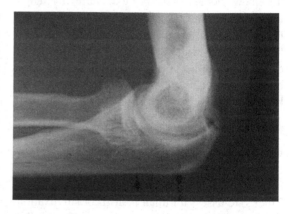

Fig. 9.4 Lateral radiograph of the elbow showing a prominent osteophyte at the tip of the olecranon. Patients who have X-ray results consistent with valgus extension overload need an MRI scan to assess the MCL (From Dodson CC, Altchek DW. The Management of Medial Collateral Ligament Tears in the Athlete. Oper Tech Sports Med: 14(2):75–80, 2006, with permission)

for Special Surgery, however, we currently use three-dimensional volumetric gradient-echo and fast spin-echo techniques, which enables thin section (<3 mm) imaging of the elbow, thus improving visualization of partial tears of the MCL and obviating the need for contrast injection [31, 32]. Partial tears can be seen on MRI scans as areas of focal interruption that do not extend through the full thickness of the ligament. Complete tears can be seen on coronal MRI scans

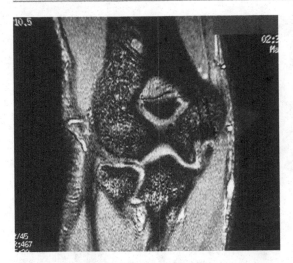

Fig. 9.5 Coronal MRI scan shows abnormal signal intensity and structure of the humeral insertion of the MCL, indicating a complete tear (From Dodson CC, Altchek DW. The Management of Medial Collateral Ligament Tears in the Athlete. Oper Tech Sports Med: 14(2):75–80, 2006, with permission)

as increased signal intensity and focal disruption of the normally hypointense, vertically oriented ligament (Fig. 9.5). In chronic ligament injuries without tears, the MCL will appear thickened without focal discontinuity, but with global increased signal intensity. Because arthroscopic evaluation of the MCL is limited in its ability to visualize the anterior bundle and humeral or ulnar insertions [25], MRI is an effective technique for distinguishing ligament tears from flexor or pronator tendinopathy. In addition, ulnar neuritis may be observed with enlargement and increased signal intensity in the nerve. Osteochondral impaction injuries to the radiocapitellar joint may also be seen, which emphasizes the importance of obtaining appropriate cartilage pulse sequencing.

Development of the Docking Procedure

Early experience of MCL reconstruction at the Hospital for Special Surgery led to some concerns about the original procedure as described by Jobe [3]. These concerns included (1) the ability to adequately tension the graft at the time of final fixation, (2) potential complications from detachment of the flexor origin, (3) potential complications from the placement of three large drill holes in a limited area on the epicondyle, (4) complications from routine ulnar nerve transposition, and (5) the strength of suture fixation of the free tendon graft. Therefore, in 1996, the senior author (DWA) began to look for alternative methods to reconstruct the MCL in order to address these concerns. The resulting procedure is referred to as the docking technique and highlights the following: (1) routine arthroscopic evaluation of the anterior and posterior compartments of the elbow to observe the degree of joint laxity and to evaluate and treat posterior medial lesions secondary to valgus extension overload, (2) using a muscle-splitting "safe zone" approach, (3) avoiding routine transposition of the ulnar nerve, (4) reducing the number of large drill holes from three to one in the medial epicondyle, and (5) addressing tendon length to ensure proper tensioning and fixation in bony tunnels [33].

Surgical Technique

At our institution, the procedure is generally performed under regional anesthesia. After the block is administered, the patient remains in the supine position, a tourniquet is placed, and the involved upper extremity is prepped and draped in the usual sterile fashion. Using an arm holder (Spider, TENET Medical Engineering, Calgary, Canada), the humerus and forearm are positioned across the patient's chest for the arthroscopic evaluation of the elbow (Fig. 9.6).

The joint is insufflated with approximately 40–50 mL of saline and an anterolateral portal is established, which facilitates arthroscopic examination of the articular surfaces and the remaining anterior compartment. An arthroscopic stress test is typically done at this point. With the elbow at 90° of flexion, the forearm is pronated and a valgus stress is applied. A positive test results in medial opening between the ulna and the humerus greater than 2 mm and is indicative of MCL insufficiency [25] (Fig. 9.7).

Fig. 9.6 The humerus and forearm are positioned across the chest and held in an arm holder to facilitate arthroscopic examination of the elbow

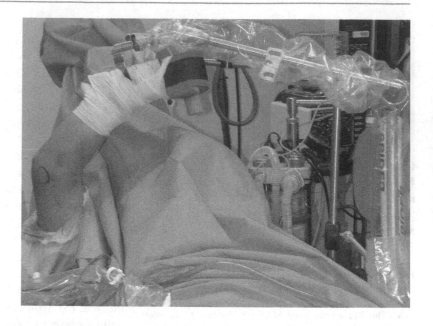

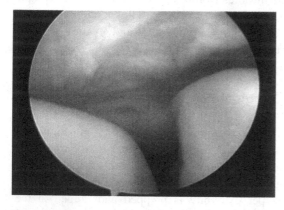

Fig. 9.7 Arthroscopic picture of a positive valgus stress test. Note the increased opening between the ulna (*left*) and the humerus (*right*), which is indicative of MCL insufficiency

After evaluating the anterior compartment, attention is then turned to the posterior compartment of the elbow. A posterolateral portal is established and the olecranon and the humeral fossae are examined for loose bodies or bone spurs. The trochlea is also examined for articular injury. Lastly, the posterior radiocapitellar joint is evaluated by advancing the arthroscope down the lateral gutter. A transtriceps portal can be created through the center of the triceps tendon at the level of the olecranon tip, which allows for

removal of loose bodies, osteophyte debridement, and microfracture of chondral lesions.

Once the arthroscopy has been completed, the arm is released from the arm holder and placed on the hand table. In cases where the palmaris longus tendon is absent, the gracilis tendon is harvested at this time. Otherwise, the ipsilateral palmaris longus tendon is harvested through a 1-cm incision in the volar wrist flexion crease over the tendon. At the time of harvest, the visible portion of the tendon is tagged with a No. 1 Ethibond suture (Ethicon, Inc., Johnson & Johnson) in a Krackow fashion and the remaining tendon is then harvested using a tendon stripper (Fig. 9.8a, b). The incision is then closed with interrupted nylon sutures and the tendon is placed in a moist sponge on the back table.

After the arm is exsanguinated to the level of the tourniquet, an 8- to 10-cm incision is created from the distal third of the intermuscular septum across the medial epicondyle to a point 2 cm beyond the sublime tubercle of the ulna. While exposing the fascia of the flexor–pronator mass, care is taken to identify and preserve the antebrachial cutaneous branch of the medial nerve, which frequently crosses the operative field. A muscle-splitting approach is then utilized through the posterior one third of the common

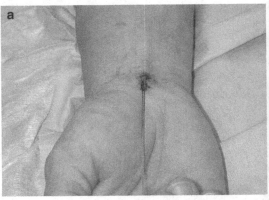

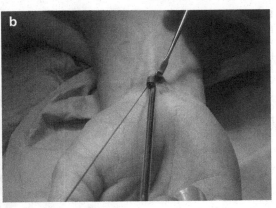

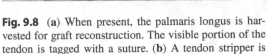

Fig. 9.8 (a) When present, the palmaris longus is harvested for graft reconstruction. The visible portion of the tendon is tagged with a suture. (b) A tendon stripper is used to harvest the remaining tendon once it has been identified and tagged

flexor pronator mass within the most anterior fibers of the FCU muscle. This approach is beneficial because it utilizes a true internervous plane, allows for adequate exposure of the native MCL, and is less traumatic than detaching the entire flexor-pronator mass from its origin [34]. The anterior bundle of the MCL is now incised longitudinally to expose the joint.

The tunnel positions for the ulna are exposed first. The posterior tunnel requires that the surgeon subperiosteally expose the ulna 4–5 mm posterior to the sublime tubercle while meticulously protecting the ulnar nerve. Using a 3-mm burr, tunnels are made anterior and posterior to the sublime tubercle such that a 2-cm bridge exists between them. The tunnels are connected using a small, curved curette, taking care not to violate the bony bridge. A suture passer is used to pass a looped suture through the tunnel. To expose the humeral tunnel position, the incision within the native MCL is extended proximally to the level of the epicondyle. A longitudinal tunnel is then created along the axis of the medial epicondyle using a 4-mm burr; care is taken not to violate the posterior cortex of the proximal epicondyle. The upper border of the epicondyle, just anterior to the intramuscular septum, is then exposed, and two small exit punctures are made with a 1.5-mm burr. They should be approximately 5 mm–1 cm apart from each other. Again a suture passer is used from each of the two exit punctures to pass a looped suture, which will be used later for graft passage. With the elbow reduced, the incision in the native MCL is repaired using a 2–0 absorbable suture.

With the forearm supinated and applying a mild varus stress to the elbow, the graft is then passed through the ulnar tunnel from anterior to posterior (Fig. 9.9). The limb of the graft on which sutures have already been placed is then passed into the humeral tunnel with the sutures exiting one of the small humeral exit punctures. This first limb of the graft is now securely "docked" in the humerus. With the elbow reduced, the graft is tensioned in flexion and extension to determine what length would be optimal by placing the second limb of the graft adjacent to the humeral tunnel. Final length is determined by referencing the graft to the exit hole in the humeral tunnel. This point is marked on the graft and a No. 1 Ethibond suture is placed in a Krackow fashion (Fig. 9.10). The excess graft is then excised immediately above the Krackow stitch and this end of the graft is then docked securely in the humeral tunnel, with the sutures exiting the free exit puncture.

Final graft tensioning is now performed by taking the elbow through a full range of motion. Once the surgeon is satisfied, the two sets of graft sutures are tied over the bony bridge on the humeral epicondyle (Fig. 9.11). After the tourniquet is deflated and hemostasis achieved, an ulnar

Fig. 9.9 The graft is passed through the ulnar tunnel from anterior to posterior. The limb of the graft with sutures is then docked into the humeral tunnel with the sutures exiting one of the exit holes

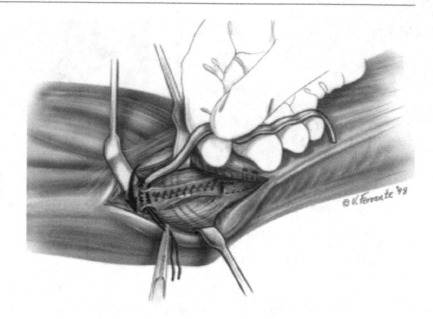

Fig. 9.10 The final length of the tendon is marked on the graft and another tagging stitch is placed (From Rohrbough et al [33])

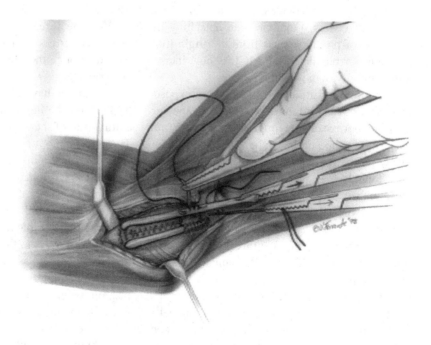

nerve transposition is performed if indicated. We only do this when the preoperative exam is consistent with ulnar neuritis. Otherwise, the fascia over the flexor pronator mass is reapproximated and the remaining wound is closed in layers. The elbow is then placed in a plaster splint at 45° of flexion and neutral rotation with the hand and wrist free.

Fig. 9.11 Once both limbs of the graft have been successfully docked into the humeral tunnel, the graft sutures are tied down (From Rohrbough et al [33])

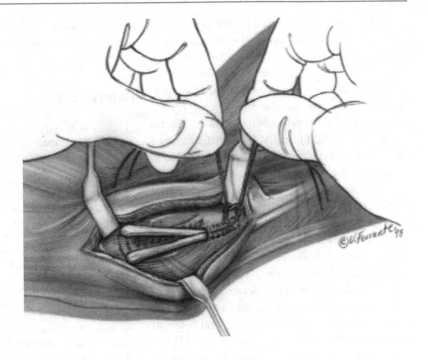

Postoperative Management

Immediately after surgery, the patients' arm is placed in a plaster splint for approximately 1 week. At the first postoperative visit, the sutures are removed and the elbow is placed in a hinged brace. Initially, motion is only allowed from 30° of extension to 90° of flexion. In the third to fifth week, motion is advanced to 15° of extension and 105° of flexion. Wrist flexion of the contralateral limb is also encouraged if the palmaris longus was harvested from that forearm. At 6 weeks, the brace is discontinued and formal physical therapy is begun, which focuses on shoulder and forearm strengthening as well as elbow range of motion. By 12 weeks, the patient is advanced to an aggressive physical therapy program that includes trunk strengthening as well as shoulder and scapula strengthening. A formal tossing program is begun at 16 weeks. Initially, throwing starts at a distance of 45 ft and is advanced at regular stages. If pain occurs during any stage, the patient is instructed to back up to the previous stage of therapy. If at 9 months the patient can throw pain free from 180 ft, they are allowed to begin pitching from a mound. We generally discourage competitive pitching until 1 year postoperatively.

Results

Conway et al [1]. conducted the first outcome study on the original procedure, as described by Jobe [3], which included detachment of the flexor–pronator mass and routine transposition of the ulnar nerve. Only 68% of the athletes in that series were able to return to either their previous or a higher level of competition. In addition, 21% of the patients were observed to develop postoperative ulnar nerve neuropathies.

Thompson and Jobe were the first to report on 83 athletes who underwent MCL reconstruction using a muscle-splitting approach without transposition of the ulnar nerve. Of these 83 patients, 33 were followed for at least 2 years. The surgical result was excellent in 27 (82%) of 33 patients, good in 4 patients (12%), and fair in 2 patients (6%). These results improved to 93% excellent when those patients who had had a prior procedure were excluded [7]. Several authors have since reported on MCL reconstruction, using a muscle-splitting approach or transposing the ulnar nerve subcutaneously, and noted lower ulnar nerve-related complication rates, ranging from 8% to 9% [35, 36].

We have recently reported on 100 consecutive MCL reconstructions using the docking technique with an average follow–up of 3 years [37]. No patients were lost to follow-up. Ninety (90%) of 100 patients returned to or exceeded their previous level of competition for at least 1 year, meeting the Conway-Jobe classification criteria of "excellent." Additionally, seven patients had a good result, which means that they were able to compete at a lower level for at least 12 months. Two patients (2%) had poor results and were not able to return to throwing.

In our series, 22% of patients underwent a subcutaneous transposition with fascial sling at the time of surgery. None of these patients suffered postoperative complications. Two athletes (2%) required transposition postoperatively after they had returned to throwing for at least 1 year. Neither patient had preoperative symptoms, and both had excellent results at the time of follow-up [37].

As previously stated, we routinely perform an arthroscopic evaluation both anteriorly and posteriorly of all patients prior to reconstruction. It is not unusual for this patient group to develop intraarticular pathology secondary to the mechanics of valgus extension overload. In our recent series, 45 (45%) of 100 patients had associated intraarticular pathology that were all managed arthroscopically just before reconstruction [37]. Detection of the lesions on preoperative imaging studies occurred in only 25 of these 45 cases. Without arthroscopy, a posterior arthrotomy is necessary to treat such pathology, which necessitates transposition of the ulnar nerve. Arthroscopy is a more minimally invasive approach and has the added benefit of avoiding obligatory transposition of the nerve. Before our use of routine arthroscopy, we had patients who required repeat surgery for conditions that were unrecognized and could have been treated arthroscopically at the time of the initial procedure.

Summary

We think that the modifications described in the "docking technique" have resulted in excellent outcomes for athletes at all levels of play and that this technique has proven to be a minimally invasive and reliable method of reconstruction of the MCL.

References

1. Conway JE, Jobe FW, Glousman RE, Pink M. Medial instability of the elbow in throwing athletes. Treatment by repair or reconstruction of the ulnar collateral ligament. J Bone Joint Surg Am 1992;74(1):67–83.
2. Hamilton CD, Glousman RE, Jobe FW, Brault J, Pink M, Perry J. Dynamic stability of the elbow: electromyographic analysis of the flexor pronator group and the extensor group in pitchers with valgus instability. J Shoulder Elbow Surg 1996;5(5):347–354.
3. Jobe FW, Stark H, Lombardo SJ. Reconstruction of the ulnar collateral ligament in athletes. J Bone Joint Surg Am 1986;68(8):1158–1163.
4. Tullos HS, Erwin WD, Woods GW, Wukasch DC, Cooley DA, King JW. Unusual lesions of the pitching arm. Clin Orthop 1972;88:169–182.
5. Waris W. Elbow injuries of javelin-throwers. Acta Chir Scand 1946;93:563–575.
6. Kenter K, Behr CT, Warren RF, O'Brien SJ, Barnes R. Acute elbow injuries in the National Football League. J Shoulder Elbow Surg 2000;(9):1–5.
7. Thompson WH, Jobe FW, Yocum LA, Pink MM. Ulnar collateral ligament reconstruction in athletes: muscle-splitting approach without transposition of the ulnar nerve. J Shoulder Elbow Surg 2001;10(2):152–157.
8. Josefsson O, Gentz CF, Johnell O, et al. Surgical versus non-surgical treatment of ligamentous injuries following dislocation of the elbow joint. J Bone Joint Surg Am 1987;69:605–608.
9. Miller CD, Savoie FH, III. Valgus Extension Injuries of the Elbow in the Throwing Athlete. J Am Acad Orthop Surg 1994;2(5):261–269.
10. Callaway GH, Field LD, Deng XH, Torzilli PA, O'Brien SJ, Altchek DW, et al. Biomechanical evaluation of the medial collateral ligament of the elbow. J Bone Joint Surg Am 1997;79(8):1223–1231.
11. Hotchkiss RN, Weiland AJ. Valgus stability of the elbow. J Orthop Res 1987;5(3):372–377.
12. Morrey BF, An KN. Articular and ligamentous contributions to the stability of the elbow joint. Am J Sports Med 1983;11(5):315–319.
13. Morrey BF, Tanaka S, An KN. Valgus stability of the elbow. A definition of primary and secondary restraints. Clin Orthop 1991;265:187–195.
14. Regan WD, Korinek SL, Morrey BF, An KN. Biomechanical study of ligaments around the elbow joint. Clin Orthop 1991;271:170–179.
15. Sojbjerg JO, Ovesen J, Nielsen S. Experimental elbow instability after transaction of the medial collateral ligament. Clin Orthop 1987;218:186–190.
16. Andrews JR, Whiteside JA. Common elbow problems in the athlete. J Orthop Sports Phys Ther 1993;17(6): 289–295.

17. Glousman RE, Barron J, Jobe FW, Perry J, Pink M. An electromyographic analysis of the elbow in normal and injured pitchers with medial collateral ligament insufficiency. Am J Sports Med 1992;20(3): 311–317.

18. Timmerman LA, Schwartz ML, Andrews JR. Preoperative evaluation of the ulnar collateral ligament by magnetic resonance imaging and computed tomography arthrography. Evaluation in 25 baseball players with surgical confirmation. Am Sports Med 1983;11(2):83–88.

19. Wilson FD, Andrews JR, Blackburn TA, McCluskey G. Valgus extension overload in the pitching elbow. Am J Sports Med 1983;11(2):83–88.

20. Fuss FK. The ulnar collateral ligament of the human elbow joint. Anatomy, function, and biomechanics. J Anat 1991;175:203–212.

21. Morrey BF, An KN. Functional anatomy of the ligaments of the elbow. Clin Orthop 1985;201:84–90.

22. O'Driscoll SW, Jaloszynski R, Morrey BF, An KN. Origin of the medial ulnar collateral ligament. J Hand Surg Am 1992;17(1):164–168.

23. Timmerman LA, Andrews JR. Undersurface tear of the ulnar collateral ligament in baseball players. A newly recognized lesion. Am J Sports Med 1994; 22(1):33–36.

24. Schwab GH, Bennett JB, Woods GW, Tullos HS. Biomechanics of elbow instability: the role of the medial collateral ligament. Clin Orthop 1980;146: 42–52.

25. Field LD, Callaway GH, O'Brien SJ, Altchek DW. Arthroscopic assessment of the medial collateral ligament complex of the elbow. Am J Sports Med 1995;23(4):396–400.

26. Davidson PA, Pink M, Perry J, Jobe FW. Functional anatomy of the flexor pronator muscle group in relation to the medial collateral ligament of the elbow. Am J Sports Med 1995;23(2):245–250.

27. O'Driscoll SW, Lawton RL, Smith AM. The "Moving Valgus Stress Test" for medial collateral ligament tears of the elbow. Am J Sports Med 2005;33(2): 231–239.

28. Ellenbecker TS, Mattalino AJ, Elam EA, Caplinger RA. Medial elbow joint laxity in professional baseball pitchers. A bilateral comparison using stress radiography. Am J Sports Med 1998;26(3):420–424.

29. Rijke AM, Goitz HT, McCue FC, Andrews JR, Berr SS. Stress radiography of the medial elbow ligaments. Radiology 1994;191(1):213–216.

30. Schwartz ML, Al Zahrani S, Morwessel RM, Andrews JR. Ulnar collateral ligament injury in the throwing athlete: evaluation with saline-enhanced MR arthrography. Radiology 1995;197(1):297–299.

31. Gaary EA, Potter HG, Altchek DW. Medial elbow pain in the throwing athlete: MR imaging evaluation. Am J Roentgenol 1997;168(3):795–800.

32. Potter HG. Imaging of posttraumatic and soft tissue dysfunction of the elbow. Clin Orthop 2000;370: 9–18.

33. Rohrbough JT, Altchek DW, Hyman J, et al. Medial collateral ligament reconstruction of the elbow using the docking technique. Am J Sports Med 2002;30(4): 541–548.

34. Smith GR, Altchek DW, Pagnani MJ, Keeley JR. A muscle-splitting approach to the ulnar collateral ligament of the elbow. Neuroanatomy and operative technique. Am J Sports Med 1996;24(5):575–580.

35. Azar FM, Andrews JR, Wilk KE, et al. Operative treatment of ulnar collateral ligament injuries of the elbow in athletes. Am J Sports Med 2000;28:16–23.

36. Elattrache NS, Bast SC, Tal D. Medial collateral ligament reconstruction. Tech Shoulder Elbow Surg 2001;2(1):38–49.

37. Dodson CC, Thomas A, Dines JS et al. Medial collateral ligament reconstruction of the elbow in throwing athletes. Am J Sports Med 2006;34:1926–1932.

Mini-incision Distal Biceps Tendon Repair

Bradford O. Parsons and Matthew L. Ramsey

Rupture of the biceps tendon from its distal insertion has historically been considered a rare injury, and early management was mainly nonoperative, with early reports citing satisfactory results [1]. However, more recent literature has recognized the persistent deficits of supination strength and endurance, and to a lesser degree flexion, in active high-demand patients, and has implicated these outcomes as an indication for acute repair [2–6]. Distal biceps ruptures currently seem to be encountered more frequently then historically reported, possibly due to increased awareness, and most surgeons now recommend early repair to maintain supination and flexion strength and endurance.

Complete distal biceps ruptures have been classified chronologically, with acute tears being recognized within 4 weeks from rupture, while chronic repairs are diagnosed after 4 weeks. With chronic tears, the integrity of the lacertus fibrosis may play a role in the degree of retraction and therefore the reparability of the tendon rupture. More recently, partial tears of the distal biceps have been recognized, and are classified by location, either insertional or intrasubstance [7–10]. Traditionally managed nonoperatively, some series have begun to elucidate the role of operative management of high-grade, symptomatic partial tears in certain patients [8].

When indicated for repair, two operative approaches are most commonly used, either a one-incision repair utilizing suture anchors or other devices to secure the biceps to the radial tuberosity, or, more commonly, a two-incision technique that utilizes a bone trough and tunnels in the tuberosity, as a modification of the original Boyd-Anderson technique [11]. Much debate has occurred in the orthopedic literature regarding one-incision versus two-incision techniques for repair of distal biceps ruptures, and numerous studies have been performed attempting to identify which approach is "better." [12–16] Proponents of the two-incision technique think that it is a stronger repair then the one-incision technique, because it reattaches the tendon directly into a bony trough. Additionally, the two-incision technique has historically been thought to have a lower likelihood of neurovascular complications [16–18]. Those who favor one-incision approaches think that the repair is as strong as the two-incision technique, but minimizes the risk of heterotopic bone and radioulnar synostosis because the tendon is not passed between the radius and ulna during repair [14, 19, 20]. Suffice it to say that the controversy still rages to some degree, and therefore we will present both the one-incision and two-incision techniques, both of which allow the use of mini-incisions to repair acute distal biceps ruptures.

B.O. Parsons (✉)
Department of Orthopaedics, Mount Sinai School of Medicine, New York, NY, USA
e-mail: bradford.parsons@mountsinai.org

G.R. Scuderi and A.J. Tria (eds.), *Minimally Invasive Surgery in Orthopedics: Upper Extremity Handbook*,
DOI 10.1007/978-1-4614-0673-0_10, © Springer Science+Business Media, LLC 2012

Pathoanatomy

Most distal biceps ruptures occur at the insertion of the tendon onto the radial tuberosity, often in the presence of preexisting tendon degeneration or partial tearing. The biceps muscle is the most anterior muscle in the anterior compartment of the arm and contributes to the formation of the lacertus fibrosis (the bicipital aponeurosis) at the level of the muscle–tendon junction. The lacertus arises off of the medial aspect of the biceps muscle and fans out across the antecubital fossa, connecting with the fascia of the proximal flexor muscles of the forearm, finally attaching to the subcutaneous border of the ulna. Deep to the lacertus, the biceps tendon travels distally to its insertion onto the radial tuberosity.

An understanding of the neurovascular structures around the elbow, especially the lateral antebrachial cutaneous nerve, median nerve, radial nerve, and posterior interosseous nerve (PIN), is critical to avoiding injury to these structures during surgical repair. The lateral antebrachial cutaneous nerve, which is the terminal sensory branch of the musculocutaneous nerve, sits lateral to the biceps tendon in the antecubital fossa. The median nerve lies medial to the biceps tendon in the antecubital fossa. The radial nerve lies between the brachialis and brachioradialis proximal to the elbow, then divides, giving off a superficial (sensory) and deep branch (PIN). The PIN dives into the supinator on the lateral side of the proximal radius, while the superficial branch sits under the brachioradialis as it travels distally into the forearm.

With complete ruptures, the biceps tendon will retract, often either to the level of the lacertus fibrosis, which if intact may tether the tendon distally, or more proximally in situations where the lacertus has been compromised. With retraction, the biceps tendon often "rolls-up" on itself, forming a ball of tendon, which, if not identified early, can degenerate, making late (>4 weeks) primary repair difficult or impossible. The biceps' tunnel (between the proximal radius and ulna) to the tuberosity is narrow, and varies in size depending upon the rotation of the forearm. In pronation, the biceps takes up 85% of the space in the tunnel, while, in supination, more space is available between the radius and ulna [21].

Diagnosing Distal Biceps Ruptures

Acute ruptures of the biceps are often made by history and physical examination. As stated, the distal biceps most frequently ruptures off of the radial tuberosity, usually during a rapid or sudden eccentric contraction of the biceps, most frequently in men around the age of 50 years. Patients often report a "pop" and immediate pain in the antecubital fossa following injury, and may develop ecchymosis after injury. Rupture often results in a deformity of the contour of the biceps muscle belly, which may be accentuated when a biceps contraction is attempted. However, in a patient with large arms, it may be difficult to clinically appreciate a muscular deformity, and therefore clinical examination is critical to the appropriate diagnosis.

Palpation of the antecubital fossa often elicits tenderness along the course of the normal biceps tendon. A defect in the fossa is indicative of a full rupture. Integrity of the lacertus fibrosis should also be assessed. As stated previously, if the lacertus is ruptured, the biceps tendon can retract further proximally. In the acute phase, pain often prohibits normal flexion of the elbow or rotation of the forearm, but as the pain and swelling subside, motion improves. Often flexion strength will be nearly equal to the contralateral side, but may elicit discomfort, or accentuate deformity of the biceps contour. Provocative testing of supination is more diagnostic. Patients with full ruptures will have weakness when asked to hold a supinated position against forceful pronation, and will also fatigue quickly as the supinator fatigues. It is important to assess cyclic strength in someone who has good strength on initial testing, as this can be helpful in identifying partial tears as well.

Radiographs are not very helpful in the diagnosis of a distal biceps rupture, as the results are most often normal. Magnetic resonance imaging (MRI) may be helpful, although not necessary in patients where history and clinical examination confirm a rupture. MRI may be used to identify partial tears, although differentiating partial tearing versus bicipital aponeurosis or tendonosis can be difficult [10]. In chronic cases, or when the history and exam do not yield an obvious diagnosis, an MRI scan can help confirm the diagnosis.

Indications for Repair

Most surgeons currently recommend surgical repair of distal biceps ruptures in the active patient [2–4, 6, 17, 22]. Once a full rupture is identified, patients should be counseled on the likely outcome of nonoperative and operative treatment. It is well established in the literature that early repair offers the best opportunity for preserving flexion and supination strength and endurance [2–4, 6, 17, 22]. Although some patients with low demands of their injured extremity may have a satisfactory outcome with nonoperative treatment, most distal biceps ruptures occur in active, middle-aged men, who often poorly tolerate the functional loss and symptoms associated with the results of nonoperative treatment. Patients who are identified acutely following rupture, especially in the first 10 days, are often amenable to a minimally invasive approach to repair [18]. However, with further delay in diagnosis, especially after 1–2 months, a more extensive dissection and exposure is required, and tendon grafts may be needed to reconstruct the tendon defect [6].

Patients with high-grade partial tears who are symptomatic and have failed nonoperative modalities including therapy are also amenable to repair of their partial tear. As awareness of this clinical entity has increased, these patients are more frequently being identified, and early reports have found successful outcomes with completion and repair of their high-grade partial biceps tears.

Contraindications

Patients who are low demand may refuse surgical repair. Additionally, patients who cannot safely undergo surgery because of medical comorbidities should be managed nonoperatively. As opposed to acute tears, patients who have chronic tears, especially those who are months removed from their injury date, may not be amenable to primary repair. With chronic tears, the biceps tendon scars and may degenerate, thereby shortening and making anatomic repair difficult or impossible. Additionally, the bicipital tunnel often fills with scar tissue, making identification difficult, which may require a more extensive exposure to identify and protect the neurovascular structures of the antecubital fossa. Rarely are these patients amenable to a "mini-incision" type of approach. Often they require an extensive exposure and tendon grafts for reconstruction.

When to Attempt Mini-incision Repairs of the Distal Biceps

Ruptures addressed within 4 weeks from injury, especially if they are within the first 2 weeks, can often be surgically repaired using mini-incisions with either a one-incision or a two-incision technique. The original Boyd–Anderson anterior incision involved a large L-shaped incision along the lateral border of the biceps proximally and a transverse distal component in the flexion crease (Fig. 10.1) [11]. This type of anterior incision is usually not necessary in the acute setting, especially when the lacertus fibrosis is intact. Often, a single transverse incision located in the flexion crease is sufficient for the anterior exposure (Fig. 10.2). If performing a two-incision technique, the anterior incision can be as small as 2 cm, but may need to be slightly wider if performing a one-incision technique (to allow additional exposure to the radial tuberosity).

Familiarity with the typical course of the biceps tendon between the radius and ulna, and its usual point of retraction when torn, helps in keeping incisions small. Typically, the biceps retracts just proximal to the flexion crease and is often more superficial than most think. The distal stump of tendon can usually be palpated proximally just beneath the skin. If there is substantial proximal retraction, as in the case of chronic tears, or where the lacertus fibrosis has been ruptured, then an L-type incision, as originally described by Boyd and Anderson, may be necessary.

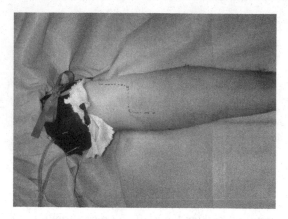

Fig. 10.1 Traditional skin incision employed in the original Boyd-Anderson technique. The proximal extent of the incision is often not necessary in acute tears. The distal extent is may be necessary for single-incision techniques

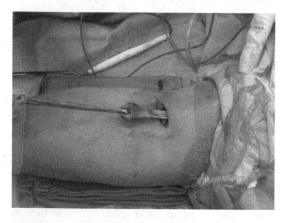

Fig. 10.2 A straight horizontal incision measuring approximately 2 cm in the anterior flexion crease is usually sufficient for identification and mobilization of acute tears

Surgical Procedure: The Two-Incision Technique

Patient Positioning

Patients are positioned supine with the affected arm on a hand table. Either regional or general anesthesia can be used. Tourniquet control may be helpful, and should be placed on the proximal arm. The tourniquet is not inflated initially, as it may inhibit excursion of the biceps tendon, and an attempt should be made to perform the repair without tourniquet inflation initially.

The extremity is draped free, and the hand covered with stockinet. The anterior incision is marked in the flexion crease of the antecubital fossa of the elbow. As stated above, a 2- to 3-cm incision is often sufficient, depending upon the size of the arm.

Instrumentation

Certain instruments and equipment are necessary to perform the two-incision technique. A bipolar cautery and standard cautery should both be available. We routinely use two #2 Fiberwire sutures (Arthrex, Naples, FL) to reattach the tendon, but any heavy, nonabsorbable suture may be used. A 2.0-mm drill bit and drill is used to make bone tunnels in the radial tuberosity, and a 3.1-mm round tip burr is used to make a trough in the tuberosity. A Hewson suture-passing device can be used to pass sutures through bone tunnels.

Procedure

Once the patient is anesthetized, positioned, and prepped and draped, a 2- to 3-cm skin incision is made in the flexion crease. Dissection is carried into the subcutaneous tissue, to the level of the deep fascia. The lateral antebrachial cutaneous nerve is identified on the lateral aspect of the incision and it should be retracted laterally. Often, a rent in the deep fascia is observed, and digital palpation will identify the bicipital tunnel to the radial tuberosity. If the fascia is intact, it should be incised and then the biceps stump should be identified. The biceps tendon will often retract to the level of the lacertus fibrosis, but may retract more proximally if the aponeurosis is torn. In most acute tears, the biceps stump can often be palpated just proximal to the incision, on the undersurface of the fascia. Once identified, the stump is passed into the wound distally, freshened, and secured with two running Krakow-type sutures utilizing #2 Fiberwire (or other stout, nonabsorbable sutures). The sutures should be cut to slightly different lengths to identify matched pairs easily once they have been passed

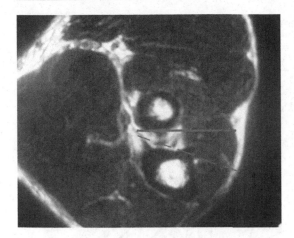

Fig. 10.3 Care is taken to develop the posterior interval (with a hemostat or other blunt instrument) around the proximal radius to the posterior aspect of the forearm (*red solid line*) so that it does not contact the ulna or disrupt the ulnar periosteum (*red dashed line*). This ensures that the posterior approach to the tuberosity is performed through a muscle-splitting approach to minimize the chance of radioulnar synostosis

posteriorly. The sutures are then clamped for later passage to the posterior incision.

As stated, the tunnel for the biceps is often easily identifiable in the acute setting. Keeping the forearm in maximal supination, the biceps tuberosity can be palpated deep in the antecubital fossa. A blunt hemostat is then passed between the radius and ulna, hugging the radial tuberosity, into the subcutaneous tissue of the posterolateral forearm (Fig. 10.3). Care must be taken to stay on the medial surface of the radius, and to not violate the ulnar periosteum, in an effort to minimize the risk of radioulnar synostosis. Once the hemostat has been passed around the radial tuberosity, the arm can be pronated, and attention turned to the posterolateral second incision.

The posterior incision utilized in a two-incision technique is also a "mini-incision." Morrey's modification of the Boyd–Anderson approach utilizes a muscle-splitting approach to minimize the chance of radioulnar synostosis (Fig. 10.3) [4]. The location of the posterior incision is identified by a hemostat passed through the radioulnar joint at the level of the radial tuberosity. The skin incision is centered over the hemostat, and usually a 3-cm skin incision is sufficient in most patients.

The incision is carried down to the fascia sharply, and then an electrocautery is used to perform a muscle-splitting approach down to the tuberosity. This is done in maximal pronation, to protect the PIN.

The superficial fascia and common extensor muscle is incised in line with the skin incision. The supinator can be identified as the fibers travel obliquely across the wound. Keeping the forearm in maximal pronation, the supinator fibers are incised over the radial tuberosity, which is often palpable at this point. The tuberosity is then exposed and cleaned of soft tissue. Self-retaining retractors are placed to keep the incision open, and small Homan retractors are placed anterior and posterior to the tuberosity. Utilizing a 3.1-mm round-tipped, high-speed burr, a 1.5-cm by 5-mm trough is made in the radial tuberosity, large enough to place the biceps tendon stump into. Using a 2.0-mm drill bit, three drill holes are made in the posterior cortex of the radial tuberosity, exiting in the bone trough, with care taken to ensure at least a 5-mm bone bridge between holes (Fig. 10.4). Copious irrigation is used to remove all bony debris, in an effort to minimize heterotopic bone formation.

The arm is then supinated, and, using a curved hemostat, the Fiberwire sutures are passed through the biceps tract, hugging the radial tuberosity, and into the posterior skin incision. Care is taken to ensure that the lateral antebrachial cutaneous nerve remains lateral to the biceps tendon at all times and does not become tethered around the tendon. The arm in pronated, and the elbow flexed to deliver the sutures posteriorly. Using a suture-passing device, the proximal limb of the proximal Krakow suture is passed through the proximal drill hole of the radial tuberosity, followed by the two middle sutures (one from each Krakow) into the middle hole, and finally the distal limb into the distal hole. Once passed, the slack is taken out of the sutures and the biceps is delivered into the bone trough. The appropriate paired sutures (identified by their slightly different lengths) are then tied over the posterior bone bridge.

At completion of the repair, the elbow is gently ranged while in supination, assessing the excursion of the repair, in an effort to guide rehabilitation. The wounds are irrigated and closed

Fig. 10.4 Once the radial tuberosity is exposed, a bony trough is made to receive the freshened tendon end. Three 2.0-mm drill holes are made along the posterior cortex of the tuberosity, with care taken to ensure an adequate bone bridge between drill holes

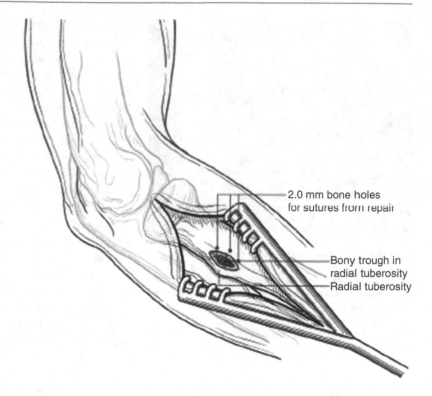

2.0 mm bone holes for sutures from repair

Bony trough in radial tuberosity
Radial tuberosity

sequentially. The anterior skin incision is closed in layers, utilizing a subcuticular stitch for the skin. If the biceps rupture is more chronic and shortening of the tendon has occurred, it may be advantageous to close the anterior skin incision after the biceps sutures have been passed posteriorly, but before they have been tied, as elbow extension and exposure to the anterior incision may be compromised. Similarly, the posterior skin incision is also closed in layers, utilizing a running subcuticular skin closure. Drains are usually not necessary. The elbow is immobilized in 90° flexion with the forearm in supination.

Surgical Procedure: The One-Incision Technique

Patient Positioning

As with the two-incision technique, patients are positioned supine, with the extremity on a hand table. A tourniquet is placed on the upper arm but often is not inflated. The arm is prepped and draped free.

Instrumentation

Many variations of the one-incision technique have been described, utilizing suture anchors, EndoButtons, pullout sutures over an external button, interference screws, etc. As such, it is beyond the scope of this text to describe all of these various techniques utilizing all of the possible fixation methods. We will describe the technique utilizing suture anchors in the radial tuberosity as an illustrative example of the one-incision technique. Any anchor single-loaded with a heavy, nonabsorbable suture is adequate, and most techniques describe using metal anchors versus bioabsorbable anchors. A high-speed burr can be used to decorticate the tuberosity in an effort to improve tendon healing to bone.

Procedure

Once the patient is anesthetized, positioned, and prepped and draped, an upside-down L incision is made, with the horizontal limb in the elbow flexion crease, and the vertical limb extending from the medial aspect of the horizontal limb along the medial volar forearm (see Fig. 10.1). As described in the two-incision technique, a proximal extension along the volar–lateral arm is often not necessary as the biceps can often be identified and pulled distally in the acute setting by palpation in the subcutaneous tissue. However, the greater the chronicity of the injury (especially after 4 weeks), the greater the likelihood that the incision will need to be extended proximal to the elbow crease (making the inverted L into an S).

After the skin incision, dissection is carried into the subcutaneous tissue, to the level of the deep fascia. The lateral antebrachial cutaneous nerve is identified on the lateral aspect of the incision and it should be retracted laterally. Often, a rent in the deep fascia is observed, and digital palpation will identify the bicipital tunnel to the radial tuberosity. If the fascia is intact, it should be incised and then the biceps stump should be identified. The biceps tendon will often retract to the level of the lacertus fibrosis, but may retract more proximally if the aponeurosis is torn. In most acute tears, the biceps stump can often be palpated just proximal to the incision, on the undersurface of the fascia. Once identified, the stump is passed into the wound distally, freshened, and secured with a traction suture. Any adhesions around the tendon are removed so as to gain maximal excursion of the tendon.

As stated, the tunnel for the biceps is often easily identifiable in the acute setting. Keeping the forearm in maximal supination, the biceps tuberosity can be palpated deep in the antecubital fossa. In the acute setting, it is often not necessary to expose the radial nerve or PIN, but often these can be gently retracted laterally. The radial recurrent vessels often overlie the tuberosity and obscure visualization, therefore necessitating ligation. The radial artery is retracted medially after ligation of the recurrent vessels. It is important to maintain excellent hemostasis for visualization. The tuberosity is then cleaned of soft tissue and a high-speed burr is used to decorticate the surface of the tuberosity to yield a bed for tendon healing. The wound is copiously irrigated to remove all bone debris in an effort to minimize the chance of heterotopic bone formation.

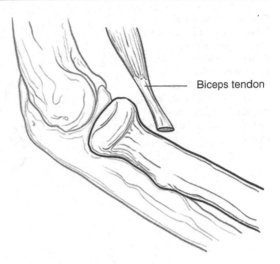

Fig. 10.5 After placement of the anchors in the radial tuberosity, the inner limb from each anchor is passed through the end of the tendon proximally in a Krakow fashion. After sufficient passage of suture, these proximal limbs are then tied together

Two suture anchors loaded with nonabsorbable sutures are then placed into the tuberosity under direct visualization in the center of the burred bed. Once placed, the anchor integrity in bone is tested and tensioned. If the anchors do not have good fixation, an alternative method of fixation may be required, such as an EndoButton, pullout sutures, tenodesis screw, etc. The inner limb of suture from each anchor is then passed into the biceps tendon in a running Krakow configuration on the respective medial and lateral aspect of the tendon. These sutures are then tied together at the proximal extent of the biceps tendon (Fig. 10.5).

Keeping the elbow flexed and the forearm in supination, the biceps tendon is delivered to the tuberosity by pulling tension on both of the remaining suture limbs (Fig. 10.6). This applies equal medial and lateral tension and brings the tendon cut surface down flush to the tuberosity bed and the anchors. Once the tendon is flush with the tuberosity bed, these two remaining suture limbs are then tied together after being appropriately tensioned. The wound is again irrigated and the integrity of the repair is evaluated to guide rehabilitation. Keeping the forearm in supination, the elbow is gently extended to test

Fig. 10.6 The distal limbs of the suture anchor can then be tightened, drawing the tendon edge into the bony bed where the anchors have been placed, and, once reduced into the bony bed, they are tied, reattaching the biceps tendon

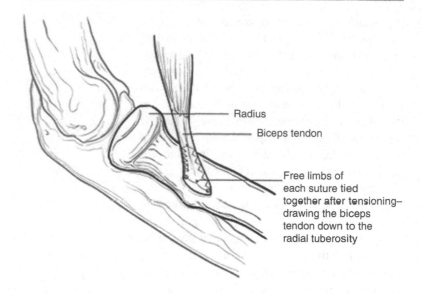

Radius

Biceps tendon

Free limbs of each suture tied together after tensioning–drawing the biceps tendon down to the radial tuberosity

the limits of range of motion. The wound is then closed in layers. Drains are usually not necessary. The elbow is immobilized in a posterior splint in maximal supination after the wound is dressed.

Postoperative Protocol

Acute repairs (within 4 weeks) are immobilized in flexion and supination in a posterior splint for 7–10 days and then the arm is placed in a hinged orthosis that maintains supination and can gradually be brought out to extension over the next few weeks. In settings where there is no tension on the repair in extension intraoperatively, the patient may be allowed to be without splint immobilization after the first postoperative visit at 7–10 days, although if any concern exists, the repair should be protected and elbow extension gradually regained. Extension is gradually regained after 8 weeks in the orthosis, following which, the patient is allowed unrestricted motion and gradual strengthening. Heavy lifting and sports are restricted until 5 months after repair.

We routinely place patients on oral indomethacin (75 mg daily) for 6 weeks following distal biceps repair to minimize the chance of heterotopic bone formation. Although the likelihood of

heterotopic ossification may be less with the one-incision technique, we would use indomethacin in these patients as well.

Results

Historical management of distal biceps ruptures was often nonoperative or nonanatomic, with mixed results. Morrey and colleagues identified some of the functional deficiencies associated with biceps ruptures, including loss of flexion and supination strength, and reported near full restoration of flexion (97%) and supination (95%) strength compared with the uninvolved extremity [4]. More recent analyses have corroborated these findings [3, 6, 17, 23]. A recent comparison of the outcome following acute repairs (<8 days) against delayed repairs (>3 weeks) found excellent results of nine patients undergoing acute repair (all of whom returned to preinjury activity levels) and nine of ten excellent results in the late repair group [6]. Outcomes were classified as excellent if flexion and supination strength was 95% of the contralateral limb, and range of motion was normal. A meta-analysis performed by the same investigators of 147 repairs found 90% excellent results following anatomic repair compared with 14% in nonoperative repairs.

Although the indication and results of acute repair have been well established, the controversy over one-incision versus two-incision techniques still rages. Numerous biomechanical studies have been performed in an attempt to identify which repair is "strongest." [13–16] Pereira and colleagues compared repairs using suture anchor repairs to bone tunnels in cadaveric specimens and found that the repair through bone tunnels was significantly stiffer and stronger, but weaker then the native tendon–bone interface [16]. Conversely, Lemos et al. found suture anchor repair using two suture anchors to be significantly stronger then bone tunnels in their biomechanical analysis (263 N vs. 203 N) [15]. Other fixation techniques have also been examined. Idler and colleagues found the failure strength and stiffness of an interference screw technique to be significantly greater then a repair through bone tunnels in cadaveric specimens [14]. Greenberg et al. reported that a repair using the EndoButton was significantly stronger then either suture anchor or bone tunnels (584 N vs. 254 N and 178 N, respectively) [13].

Although these studies shed some light on repair strength and options available for fixation, the use of cadaveric specimens for biomechanical testing has some inherent flaws, such as bone quality. Therefore, it is important to take the data in proper context. Until a randomized, prospective trial comparing one-incision to two-incision technique has shown conclusive data, either approach is a viable option when repairing a distal biceps rupture.

Complications

Early reports of the original Boyd–Anderson two-incision repairs found an unacceptable incidence of heterotopic ossification and radioulnar synostosis [4, 24]. Other early reports highlighted some of the neurovascular complications that occurred following anterior single-incision repairs, including median and radial nerve palsy. [18, 25–27]

A recent study by Kelly and colleagues at the Mayo Clinic reviewed the complication rate of 74 consecutive biceps repairs (acute, subacute, and delayed) using a modified two-incision technique [18]. The overall complication rate was 31% and included five sensory nerve paresthesias (three lateral antebrachial cutaneous, two superficial radial nerve), one PIN palsy (resolved), six patients with anterior-based elbow pain, and four cases of anterior heterotopic ossification. No patients developed radioulnar synostosis. Interestingly, the rate of neurologic complication in this series was similar to the rate following one-incision repairs.

The authors found when they subdivided acute (<10 days) from subacute (10 days to 3 weeks) and delayed (>3 weeks), the likelihood of complications was significantly greater in patients with subacute and delayed repairs. In fact, all patients with postoperative paresthesias were subacute or delayed repairs requiring a formal extended anterior Henry approach. As a result, they concluded that delayed repairs often require more extensive exposure, potentially placing neurovascular and other structures at greater risk.

Conclusion

Rupture of the distal biceps from its insertion on the radial tuberosity often leads to disability and weakness of supination and flexion of the involved extremity. Surgical repair, especially in the acute setting, has been found to reliably reestablish strength and function in the extremity. As such, most authors currently advocate acute surgical repair, although the choice of approach remains controversial. As with most other aspects of orthopedic surgery, a push has been made to perform more minimally invasive techniques for a multitude of conditions, and distal biceps ruptures are no different. The patient with an acute tear, especially those within 10 days from injury, often can be treated with a minimally invasive repair utilizing either a one-incision or a two-incision technique, depending upon surgeon preference.

References

1. Kron SD, Satinsky VP. Avulsion of the distal biceps brachii tendon. Am J Surg 1954;88(4):657–9
2. Baker BE, Bierwagen D. Rupture of the distal tendon of the biceps brachii. Operative versus non-operative treatment. J Bone Joint Surg Am 1985;67(3):414–7
3. D'Alessandro DF, Shields CL, Jr, Tibone JE, Chandler RW. Repair of distal biceps tendon ruptures in athletes. Am J Sports Med 1993;21(1):114–9
4. Morrey BF, Askew LJ, An KN, Dobyns JH. Rupture of the distal tendon of the biceps brachii. A biomechanical study. J Bone Joint Surg Am 1985;67(3): 418–21
5. Ramsey ML. Distal biceps tendon injuries: diagnosis and management. J Am Acad Orthop Surg 1999;7(3):199–207
6. Rantanen J, Orava S. Rupture of the distal biceps tendon. A report of 19 patients treated with anatomic reinsertion, and a meta-analysis of 147 cases found in the literature. Am J Sports Med 1999;27(2):128–32
7. Bourne MH, Morrey BF. Partial rupture of the distal biceps tendon. Clin Orthop Relat Res 1991;(271): 143–8
8. Kelly EW, Steinmann S, O'Driscoll SW. Surgical treatment of partial distal biceps tendon ruptures through a single posterior incision. J Shoulder Elbow Surg 2003;12(5):456–61
9. Norman WH. Repair of avulsion of insertion of biceps brachii tendon. Clin Orthop Relat Res 1985;(193): 189–94
10. Rokito AS, McLaughlin JA, Gallagher MA, Zuckerman JD. Partial rupture of the distal biceps tendon. J Shoulder Elbow Surg 1996;5(1):73–5
11. Boyd HaA, LD. A method for reinsertion of the distal biceps brachii tendon. J Bone Joint Surg Am 1961;43: 1041–3
12. Berlet GC, Johnson JA, Milne AD, Patterson SD, King GJ. Distal biceps brachii tendon repair. An in vitro biomechanical study of tendon reattachment. Am J Sports Med 1998;26(3):428–32
13. Greenberg JA, Fernandez JJ, Wang T, Turner C. EndoButton-assisted repair of distal biceps tendon ruptures. J Shoulder Elbow Surg 2003;12(5):484–90
14. Idler CS, Montgomery WH, III, Lindsey DP, Badua PA, Wynne GF, Yerby SA. Distal biceps tendon repair: a biomechanical comparison of intact tendon and 2 repair techniques. Am J Sports Med 2006;34(6): 968–74
15. Lemos SE, Ebramzedeh E, Kvitne RS. A new technique: in vitro suture anchor fixation has superior yield strength to bone tunnel fixation for distal biceps tendon repair. Am J Sports Med 2004;32(2):406–10
16. Pereira DS, Kvitne RS, Liang M, Giacobetti FB, Ebramzadeh E. Surgical repair of distal biceps tendon ruptures: a biomechanical comparison of two techniques. Am J Sports Med 2002;30(3):432–6
17. El-Hawary R, Macdermid JC, Faber KJ, Patterson SD, King GJ. Distal biceps tendon repair: comparison of surgical techniques. J Hand Surg (Am) 2003;28(3): 496–502
18. Kelly EW, Morrey BF, O'Driscoll SW. Complications of repair of the distal biceps tendon with the modified two-incision technique. J Bone Joint Surg Am 2000; 82-A(11):1575–81
19. Lintner S, Fischer T. Repair of the distal biceps tendon using suture anchors and an anterior approach. Clin Orthop Relat Res 1996;(322):116–9
20. Sotereanos DG, Pierce TD, Varitimidis SE. A simplified method for repair of distal biceps tendon ruptures. J Shoulder Elbow Surg 2000;9(3):227–33
21. Seiler JG, III, Parker LM, Chamberland PD, Sherbourne GM, Carpenter WA. The distal biceps tendon. Two potential mechanisms involved in its rupture: arterial supply and mechanical impingement. J Shoulder Elbow Surg 1995;4(3):149–56
22. Louis DS, Hankin FM, Eckenrode JF, Smith PA, Wojtys EM. Distal biceps brachii tendon avulsion. A simplified method of operative repair. Am J Sports Med 1986;14(3):234–6
23. McKee MD, Hirji R, Schemitsch EH, Wild LM, Waddell JP. Patient-oriented functional outcome after repair of distal biceps tendon ruptures using a single-incision technique. J Shoulder Elbow Surg 2005;14(3): 302–6
24. Failla JM, Amadio PC, Morrey BF, Beckenbaugh RD. Proximal radioulnar synostosis after repair of distal biceps brachii rupture by the two-incision technique. Report of four cases. Clin Orthop Relat Res 1990; (253):133–6
25. Dobbie R. Avulsion of the lower biceps brachii tendon. Analysis of fifty-one previously unreported cases. Am J Surg 1941;51:662–83
26. Friedmann E. Rupture of the distal biceps brachii tendon. Report on 13 cases. JAMA 1963;184:60–3
27. Meherin JH, Kilgore BS Jr. The treatment of ruptures of the distal biceps brachii tendon. Am J Surg 1960;99:636–40

Minimally Invasive Approaches for Complex Elbow Trauma

11

Raymond A. Klug, Jonathon Herald, and Michael R. Hausman

The use of arthroscopic approaches in complex elbow trauma has several advantages over more traditional open approaches. Arthroscopy results in less soft tissue dissection and may reduce post-operative pain and ease rehabilitation. Additionally, arthroscopy allows for improved visualization of intraarticular fractures and may improve anatomic reduction of the articular surface. Aside from standard diagnostic or therapeutic arthroscopy, there are several indications for arthroscopy in addressing fractures about the elbow.

Indications

The indications are pediatric lateral condyle fractures, coronoid fractures without associated radial head fractures, capitellum fractures, and radial head fractures. In our institution, we routinely use arthroscopy in the treatment of all of these indications with the exception of radial head fractures because we think this a technically more demanding procedure with increased risk for neurovascular injury. The following chapter focuses on arthroscopic treatment of coronoid fractures, pediatric lateral condyle fractures, and fractures of the capitellum.

Arthroscopically Assisted Treatment of Coronoid Fractures

The coronoid process of the ulna is of critical importance to elbow stability [1–7]. Although occasionally isolated injuries, fractures of the coronoid most commonly occur in association with ligamentous injury and result in varying degrees of elbow instability. The Regan and Morrey classification described three types of coronoid fractures based on the level of coronoid detachment in the coronal plane [8]. Type III fractures involve more than 50% of the coronoid process and require open reduction and internal fixation to avoid recurrent elbow instability from loss of bony constraint [8]. More recently, it has been recognized that late elbow instability resulting from soft tissue damage may occur with smaller fracture fragments and that these injuries may be more complex than previously thought (Fig. 11.1) [1, 6, 7].

In patients with apparently isolated type I or II coronoid fractures who have had computed tomography (CT) scans, we have noted the presence of a "sag sign" in the ulnohumeral joint that may be indicative of ligamentous injury due to an associated lateral ulnar collateral ligament (LUCL) or medial collateral ligament (MCL) injury resulting in posterolateral or posteromedial "sagging" of the elbow joint (Fig. 11.2) [7]. Additionally, other authors have appreciated the complexity of injury patterns associated with smaller coronoid fractures; open reduction and

M.R. Hausman (✉)
Department of Orthopaedics, Mount Sinai School of Medicine, New York, NY, USA
e-mail: michael.hausman@mountsinai.org

G.R. Scuderi and A.J. Tria (eds.), *Minimally Invasive Surgery in Orthopedics: Upper Extremity Handbook*,
DOI 10.1007/978-1-4614-0673-0_11, © Springer Science+Business Media, LLC 2012

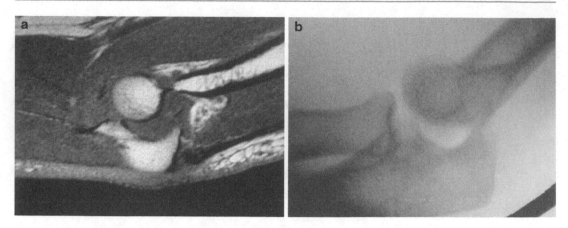

Fig. 11.1 Nonconcentric reduction of ulnohumeral joint with type I coronoid fracture suggesting additional capsulo-ligamentous injury. (**a**) MRI scan. (**b**) Fluoroscopic examination

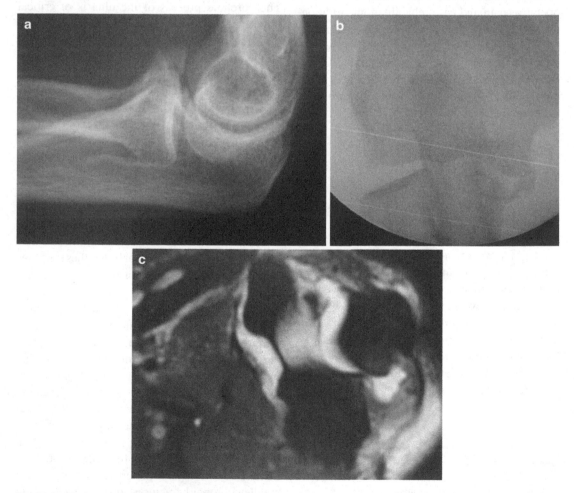

Fig. 11.2 Static varus instability in a patient with type II coronoid fracture. (**a**) Lateral view. (**b**) Anteroposterior (AP) view. (**c**) Axial MRI scan showing posteromedial subluxation

internal fixation techniques are being performed more frequently for type I and II fractures as associated elbow instability is being recognized more often [2, 3].

Persistent elbow instability is a challenging problem. Treatment of gross instability, such as that associated with a "terrible triad" type of injury, may require fixation of the coronoid and repair of the anterior capsule, as repair or reconstruction of the radial head and collateral ligaments alone may not adequately stabilize the elbow [1, 7]. Although recurrent frank dislocation is uncommon following surgical treatment of these injuries, lesser degrees of instability may result in premature degenerative changes. Fixation of the coronoid, capsular repair, and stabilization of the joint could potentially decrease this complication, although compelling evidence for this is currently lacking.

The combination of small fracture fragments, comminution, and soft tissue stripping may result in marginal fixation and residual instability despite open reduction. Additionally, there may be loss of the capsule as a stabilizing structure. A less invasive approach achieving accurate reduction and stable fixation may be advantageous when operative fracture treatment is indicated. Repair of the anterior capsule may also be important, particularly when the coronoid fragment is small or comminuted.

Indications

Doornberg and Ring suggest that Regan-Morrey type I or II coronoid fractures may be associated with a more guarded prognosis than type III fractures because the former are usually, if not always, associated with capsular disruption and/or ligamentous injury. This is not typically the case with type III fractures, which are more commonly purely bony injuries without associated ligamentous disruption [1, 9].

Various methods of coronoid and capsular repair are available. Medial coronoid compression fractures may be fixed by a medial approach and use of small screws and plates (Fig. 11.3) [7]. Larger fragments, such as the type III injury associated with a Monteggia-type fracture-dislocation,

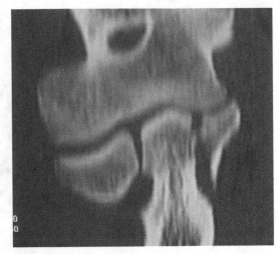

Fig. 11.3 Medial coronoid fracture

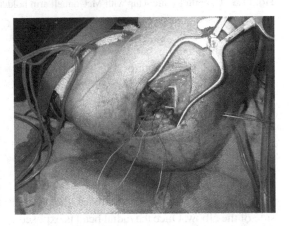

Fig. 11.4 Lateral approach after radial head removal showing capsular repair sutures being passed with a Hewson suture passer

may be reduced and fixed from the posterior approach [10]. "Terrible triad" injuries frequently necessitate radial head arthroplasty. In these cases, the coronoid and anterior capsule are accessible from the lateral approach once the radial head is removed (Fig. 11.4).

Conventional open reduction and internal fixation requires extensive exposure and frequently, detachment of residual anterior capsular attachments [3, 4]. With open approaches, a portion of the anterior capsule is detached from the proximal ulna to facilitate exposure of the fracture site. This is technically difficult and may jeopardize the vascularity of the fracture fragment. More difficult to treat are coronoid fractures with

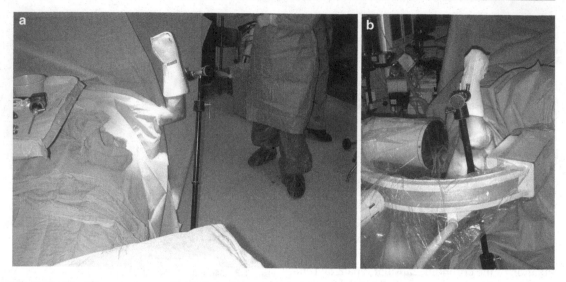

Fig. 11.5 Operating suite setup with McConnell arm holder (**a**) and Mini C-arm (**b**)

demonstrable, but lesser degrees of instability without radial head fractures or with fracture patterns less amenable to open reduction and internal fixation. In such cases, coronoid repair may be desirable, but repair by open means would require a more extensive surgical approach than would otherwise be needed (Fig. 11.4). The most relevant example of this is the "terrible triad" injury in which fracture of the radial head essentially necessitates open exposure of the lateral side of the elbow. Once the radial head is exposed, it can be retracted or removed to facilitate approach to the coronoid. Without fracture of the radial head, open exposure may no longer be necessary. In such situations, arthroscopically assisted reduction may be of greatest benefit, as it permits fixation of the coronoid and capsular repair without an otherwise unnecessary extensive surgical approach. In addition, repair of small or multiple fragments may only be feasible by capsular repair and this may be technically more feasible by arthroscopic means in those patients not requiring radial head resection for arthroplasty.

Operative Technique

Patient Positioning

The procedure is performed under nondepolarizing general or regional anesthesia. Patients are placed in the supine position with the affected arm in an arm support (McConnell arm holder, McConnell Orthopaedic Manufacturing Company, Greenville, TX) (Fig. 11.5). The involved extremity is draped free. The shoulder of the involved extremity is positioned at the edge of the bed so that the remainder of the arm can hang free over the edge. The main tube of the C-arm is sterilely draped so that the upper arm and elbow can lie on the base of C-arm, which serves as the operating table.

Arthroscopic Reduction

After marking the major landmarks and confirming the location of the ulnar nerve, a standard proximal anteromedial viewing portal is created using a blunt technique. Low infusion pressures of 25–30 mmHg are used to avoid excessive fluid extravasation. Under arthroscopic visualization, an anterolateral working portal is created and a cannula is introduced into the elbow joint. The anterior compartment of the elbow is inspected first, and a 4.5-mm shaver is used to remove any clot or fracture debris. The coronoid fragment is then visualized and the fracture site is prepared using the soft tissue shaver (Fig. 11.6g). Intraarticular retractors can be used to help with exposure. A trial reduction of the fracture fragment is attempted using an arthroscopic grasper through the anterolateral portal (Fig. 11.6h).

Fig. 11.6 Case example: 53-year-old woman with type II coronoid fracture, posteromedial subluxation, and varus instability. (**a**) Preoperative coronal CT scan showing type II fracture. (**b**) Sagittal cut showing fracture fragments and ulnohumeral subluxation. (**c**) Axial cut showing ulnohumeral subluxation. (**d**) Preoperative fluoroscopic examination. (**e**) Sagittal MRI scan. (**f**) Coronal MRI scan showing intact lateral ulnar collateral ligament. (**g**) Arthroscopic view of fracture site with hematoma. (**h**) Fracture reduction held with arthroscopic grasper. (**i**) Fluoroscopic view of guide wire placement. (**j**) Reduction held with arthroscopic clamp during drilling and screw placement. (**k**) Arthroscopic monitoring of guide wire placement. (**l**) Placement of capsular repair suture. (**m**) Intraoperative AP view showing fracture reduction and screw placement. (**n**) Intraoperative lateral view showing reduction and screw placement. (**o**) Patient range of motion 6 weeks after surgery

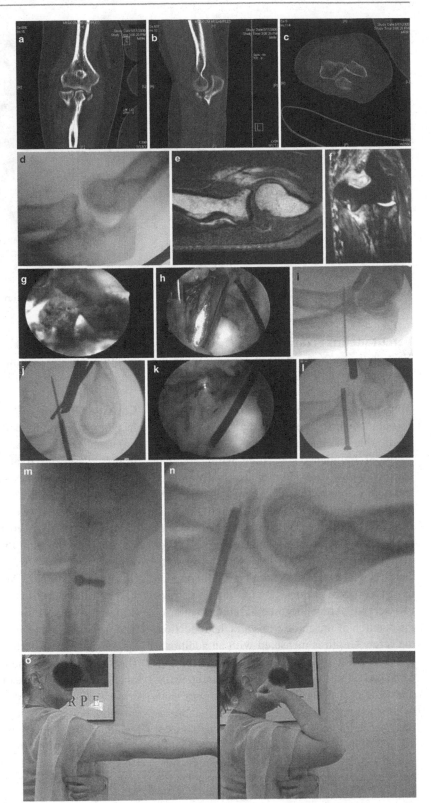

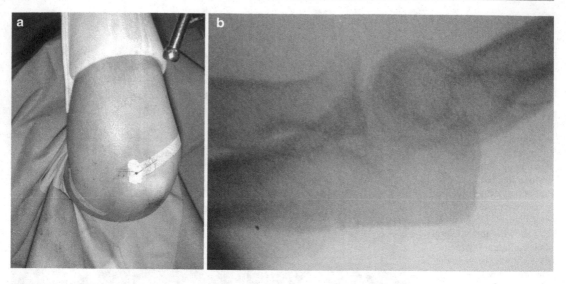

Fig. 11.7 (a) Pull-out suture placed for capsular repair. (b) Reduction is confirmed fluoroscopically

Percutaneous Fixation

Next, a 1- to 2-cm incision is made over the posterior aspect of the proximal ulna. Under fluoroscopic control, two guide pins are advanced from the posterior ulnar shaft into the base of the coronoid. Arthroscopic visualization is used to ensure that one guide wire exits centrally in the coronoid fragment. The guide wires are then backed out, and the fracture anatomically reduced and held with an arthroscopic grasper. The wires are then advanced into the coronoid fragment (Fig. 11.6i). The central wire is used for cannulated screw placement while the other wire is for derotational purposes. If the fragment is sufficiently large, two screws may be used, although most type I or II fractures are too small to accept two screws. After fluoroscopic confirmation of the position of the guide wires and the reduction, the screw length is measured with an additional identical guide wire. The original wires are then advanced slightly to avoid inadvertent withdrawal after drilling. If necessary, the wires can be grasped with an alligator clamp for stabilization. A cannulated 2.5-mm drill and tap are used and a 3.5- or 4.0-mm, short threaded cannulated screw is placed while anatomic reduction is monitored under arthroscopic visualization (Fig. 11.6k). An arthroscopic grasper or small gynecological ring curette is used to help reduce and hold the coronoid fragment or fragments in position during drilling and screw placement (Fig. 11.6j).

Capsular Repair

In type I or comminuted fractures, the coronoid fragment may be too small for screw placement. In these cases, the fixation is done with pull-out mattress sutures tied posterolaterally. To do this, an arthroscopic suture passing instrument is used to pass one or two 2–0 Proline (Ethicon, Somerville, NJ) or Fiberwire (Arthrex, Naples, FL) sutures through the anterior capsule and around the coronoid fragments. We have used the Opus suture system (ArthroCare Corp., Austin, TX) and the Spectrum soft tissue repair system (Linvatech Corp., Largo, FL) to place the sutures. Once placed, a Hewson suture retriever or a looped suture is inserted to retrieve the sutures. The sutures are then tied over the posterior, subcutaneous border of the ulna and reduction is confirmed radiographically (Fig. 11.7). This technique can also be used to augment the screw fixation techniques described above. In this case, suture retrieval is done through the cannulated screws (Fig. 11.6l). Postoperatively, all patients are immobilized in a splint for 2–3 weeks and then gradually started with physical therapy for range of motion.

Results

Preliminary results in our institution have been encouraging. In a study of four consecutive patients with Regan–Morrey type I or 2 coronoid fractures evaluated at a mean of 23.7 weeks, anatomic reduction was achieved in all patients, and all patients went on to osseous union by 6 weeks postoperatively. At final follow-up, all patients had full flexion; three patients had full extension and one patient lacked 10°. The average range of motion was 2.5–140°, with full pronation/supination. There was no residual or recurrent instability, neurovascular injury, infection, or other complications. Stress testing showed no residual varus, valgus, posteromedial, or posterolateral instability. Fluoroscopic examination revealed no instability throughout the range of motion. One patient who did not undergo screw fixation had subsequent removal of a prominent Fiberwire suture over the subcutaneous border of the ulna. One other patient complained of a prominent screw head on the subcutaneous border of the ulna, but opted against hardware removal.

Arthroscopically Assisted Treatment of Pediatric Lateral Humeral Condyle Fractures

Fractures and dislocations about the elbow are second in frequency only to distal forearm injuries in children [11]. Specifically, lateral humeral condyle fractures account for up to 17% of elbow fractures in children [12, 13].

Pediatric lateral humeral condyle fractures were classified by Milch [13] as type I or II based on the position of the fracture line in relation to the trochlear groove. Salter and Harris [14] further classified those fractures that exit medial to the trochlear groove as type IV according to their classification scheme. Nondisplaced Milch type I fractures can be treated nonoperatively; however, in our experience, truly nondisplaced fractures are rare. Type I fractures with intraarticular displacement, and all type II fractures require anatomic reduction of the articular surface.

Currently, anatomic reconstitution of the joint surface is done percutaneously following arthrography. If anatomic reduction of the joint surface cannot be achieved with this method, an open Kocher approach to the lateral side of the distal humerus is required. Open approaches not only require dissection of the fine capsulosynovial attachments, but also elevation of the periosteum of the distal fragment, both of which can compromise the vascularity of the distal fragment and lead to avascular necrosis. Arthroscopic reduction of the lateral condyle fracture may avoid this catastrophic complication while still obtaining an anatomic articular reduction. The fracture is then percutaneously pinned and immobilized for 4–6 weeks, per the standard treatment protocol.

Elbow arthroscopy can be performed safely and effectively in the pediatric population by experienced small joint arthroscopists. Micheli et al. have reported the diagnostic and therapeutic benefits of elbow arthroscopy in athletically active pediatric patients [15]. Of their 49 patients, none experienced nerve injury, infection, or postoperative loss of motion. Additionally, Dunn et al. reported good results using arthroscopic synovectomy to reduce hemarthroses in various joints including the elbow for hemophilic joint disease in the pediatric population [16].

Complications of lateral condyle fractures include avascular necrosis and cubitus valgus deformity. Avascular necrosis, often seen in cases treated with late open reduction is likely due to the extensive soft tissue dissection necessary in healed or partially healed malunited fractures [17, 18]. The primary blood supply to the lateral condyle is a branch of the radial recurrent artery entering along the posterior aspect of the distal humerus. This branch is commonly disrupted by fracture of the lateral condyle. A secondary blood supply arises from the anterolateral capsule and the synovial fold along the lateral border of the capitellum and may be injured during surgical approach. As a result, avascular necrosis may occur with fragmentation of the capitellum and lateral condyle, resulting in permanent deformity. Regardless of the presence of avascular necrosis, cubitus valgus deformity may occur as a result of

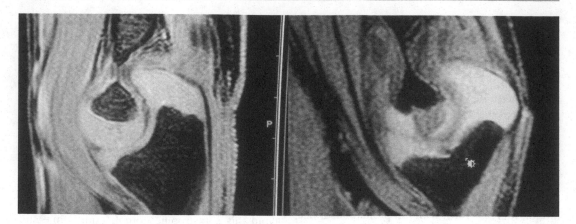

Fig. 11.8 MRI scan showing cartilaginous contribution to the elbow joint and intimate relationship of soft tissue attachments to the distal humerus

fracture malunion or less commonly secondary to lateral condylar epiphysiodesis.

Indications

Although nonoperative treatment can be considered for nondisplaced Milch I fractures, articular surface incongruity must be ruled out. This can be confirmed by arthrogram or possibly via computer tomography. If displaced or unstable fractures are treated nonoperatively, nonunion or malunion may ensue. Operative fixation is indicated in Milch II fractures, as well as displaced Milch I fractures. Great care must be taken to ensure that anatomic reduction is obtained to prevent development of irregularity at the articular surface. Because these fractures involve the physis, nonanatomic reduction may also result in complete or partial growth arrest and/or late deformity [19].

In order to ensure anatomic articular reduction, most surgeons have resorted to open approaches for displaced lateral humeral condyle fractures. Although great care is taken to preserve the posteriorly based blood supply to the capitulum, the dissection involves detachment of capsulosynovial structures and periosteum that are critical to the vascularity of the distal fracture fragment. These technical difficulties may contribute to the etiology of nonunion, malunion, valgus angulation, and avascular necrosis (Fig. 11.8) [20].

Operative Technique

Patient Positioning

The procedure is performed under nondepolarizing general anesthesia in all patients. The patients are positioned supine with the involved extremity draped free. The shoulder of the involved extremity is positioned at the edge of the bed so that the remainder of the arm can hang free over the edge. The main tube of the C-arm is sterilely draped so that the upper arm and elbow can lie on the base of the C-arm, which serves as the operating table.

Arthroscopic Reduction

After sterile preparation and draping of the involved upper extremity, standard landmarks for elbow arthroscopy are carefully marked, including the ulnar nerve and the medial epicondyle. A number 15 blade is used to incise the skin and establish a standard anteromedial portal. An atraumatic technique that involves only incision to the dermis with subcutaneous spreading to protect the cutaneous sensory nerves and a special, blunt trocar to enter the joint is used. The joint is usually distended by fracture hematoma and easily entered. A 2.5-mm wrist arthroscope is used for smaller patients (usually below age 3 years), while a standard 4.5-mm arthroscope is used beyond this age. After irrigation of the fracture hematoma, an anterolateral portal is established and used to insert a 3.5-mm shaver to

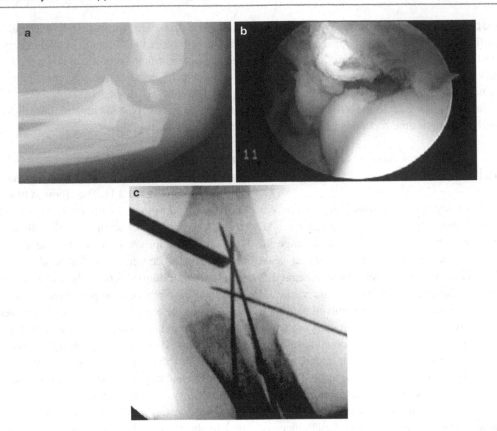

Fig. 11.9 Case example. (**a**) Preoperative lateral view showing subtle displacement of lateral condyle fracture. (**b**) Arthroscopic view showing intraarticular extension of lateral condyle fracture. (**c**) Intraoperative view showing pin placement. Note lateral to medially placed transverse pin

further debride and facilitate visualization of the fracture site. Identification of landmarks on the lateral side is difficult and the lateral portal, if necessary, is made under arthroscopic visualization from the inside–out to avoid erroneous placement.

Percutaneous Pinning

Once the fracture line is visualized, the distal fragment is anatomically reduced under arthroscopic visualization. Manual pressure over the lateral condyle is used to reduce the fracture and 0.062 K-wires are used as joysticks. Any interposed soft tissue blocking the reduction may be debrided or extracted from the fracture site using a probe, an arthroscopic grasper, or a shaver. Then, 0.062 K-wires are inserted into the lateral condyle fragment in a retrograde manner. Two

K-wires are placed in the distal–lateral portion of the fragment and advanced proximally and medially, engaging the medial cortex proximal to the fracture in a standard fashion. A third K-wire is placed at the level of the center of rotation of the capitellum in a lateral to medial direction. This wire is inserted into the trochlea transversely, in a trajectory similar to that employed in fixation of an adult intercondylar fracture, and serves three purposes regarding rotation. First, it allows visualization of the degree of rotational correction needed. Second, it is used to help derotate the fragment, and third, it allows improved fixation stability by preventing rotation around the retrograde wires (Fig. 11.9). The position and trajectory of the K-wires is confirmed fluoroscopically while maintenance of anatomic articular reduction is confirmed arthroscopically.

Postoperative Management

All patients are placed in a long arm cast postoperatively for 4–6 weeks. Patients are followed weekly with radiographs to ensure maintenance of reduction for the first 6 weeks postoperatively. The pins and cast are removed at 4 weeks postoperatively, at which time motion is begun.

Results

Preliminary results in six consecutive patients at our institution have been encouraging. All patients had full active and passive range of motion of the involved elbow from at least 5–130°. There was no statistically significant difference in flexion, extension, or arc range of motion compared with the uninvolved side ($p < 0.05$). There was no difference in carrying angle between the involved and uninvolved sides ($p < 0.05$). One patient had a slight lateral prominence. All patients were pain free at final evaluation. All fractures healed radiographically by 4 weeks. There were no cases of nonunion or malunion. One patient developed radiolucency of the capitulum, which may represent avascular necrosis.

Arthroscopically Assisted Treatment of Capitellum Fractures

Capitellar fractures may be deceptively severe; injuries and complications such as avascular necrosis, malunion, and nonunion may be more common than previously appreciated.

Operative Technique

Patient Positioning

The procedure is performed under nondepolarizing general anesthesia in all patients. The patients are positioned supine with the involved extremity draped free. The shoulder of the involved extremity is positioned at the edge of the bed so that the remainder of the arm can hang free over the edge. The main tube of the C-arm is sterilely draped so that the upper arm and elbow can lie on the base of C-arm, which serves as the operating table. The upper extremity is draped over the chest of the patient for screw placement and lateral fluoroscopic views (Fig. 11.10).

Fracture Reduction

Fracture reduction can usually be performed by closed means (Fig. 11.11). The elbow is placed in extension and pronated with a varus stress. If the fragment is reduced, the elbow is then flexed and the forearm supinated to "lock" the capitellar fragment in place with the radial head.

If the capitellum does not reduce in extension or the radial head remains too prominent to ride over the edge of the capitellar fragment, the capitellum may be manipulated using a 0.062 K-wire joystick. Arthroscopic visualization is rarely necessary at this point. If reduction cannot be achieved, a proximal anteromedial portal can be made for debridement of the hematoma with a curette. Once this is done, a posterior portal can be established proximal to the displaced capitellum. This should be done with great care as distortion of the anatomy may place the radial nerve at increased risk.

One common source of trouble is "plastic deformation" of the distal part of the lateral condyle that prevents anatomic reduction of the displaced coronoid fragment, resulting in an ovoid-shaped capitellum, rather than the desired sphere. Sagittal cuts on a limited CT scan may help anticipate this problem. If present, preliminary curettage of the posterior capitellum from a "soft spot" portal and compaction molding with a Frier or small Cobb elevator may be necessary (Fig. 11.12).

Once preliminary reduction is achieved, standard anteromedial and anterolateral portals are established and debridement is completed. The fracture line through the articular surface is the best indicator of the accuracy of reduction, and intraoperative fluoroscopy cannot always discriminate residual superior and anterior displacement of the distal edge of the capitellum.

Fig. 11.10 Typical setup of the operating room for arthroscopic reduction and internal fixation (ARIF) of a capitellum fracture. (**a**) Arthroscopic reduction and pin placement. (**b**) Drilling over cannulated wires. (**c**) Fluoroscopic evaluation of guide wire position

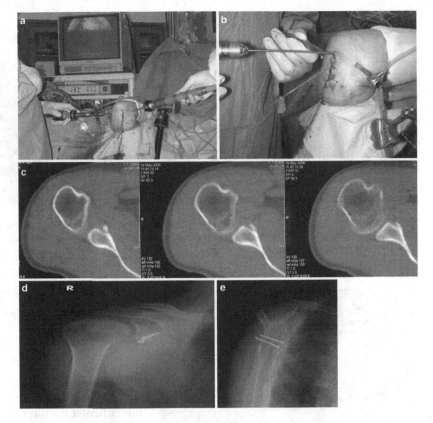

Fracture Fixation

Once accuracy of the reduction is confirmed, guide wires are inserted in a posterior to anterior direction into the capitellum for cannulated screw placement. A minimum of two screws should be used. An elevator or trochar should be inserted in the radiocapitellar joint to maintain compression across the fracture site as the wires are advanced (Fig. 11.13).

After measuring the required screw length, the wires are advanced into the radial head to prevent inadvertent extraction. The 2.5-mm cannulated drill is used, taking care not to penetrate the subchondral bone, and short threaded 3.5- or 4-mm cannulated screws are inserted. The reduction is checked once again with the arthroscope and the elbow is extended to ensure the articular surface has not been violated (Fig. 11.14).

Headed screws are utilized to take advantage of the additional support and purchase afforded

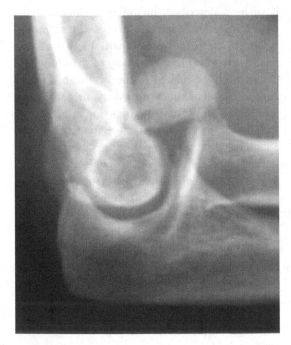

Fig. 11.11 Lateral view of a typical displaced capitellum fracture

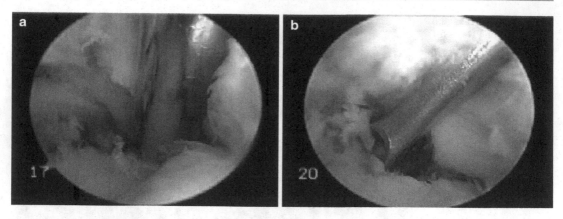

Fig. 11.12 (**a**) Malreduction of the distal edge of the capitellum is seen in this view from the posterolateral portal, passing the arthroscope down the lateral gutter. (**b**) A curette is used to remove debris blocking anatomic reduction

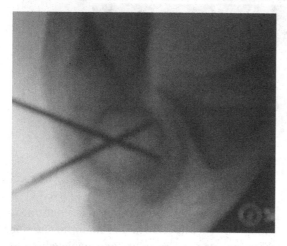

Fig. 11.13 Placement of guide wires. The screws may cross or be placed parallel to one another. The first screw should be placed distal to proximal to compress the fracture site and help reduce any residual displacement of the fragment

by cortical bone posteriorly. This is particularly important when there is only a thin shell of posterior bone. Thin anterior osteochondral fragments remain challenging even with anterior to posterior screws and may be best treated by immobilization to allow some healing and subsequent arthroscopic release of any residual contracture, rather than risking loss of a substantial portion of the articular surface. Postoperatively, all patients are immobilized in a splint for 2–3 weeks and then gradually started with physical therapy for range of motion.

Summary

Intraarticular fractures about the elbow are often difficult injuries to treat. Several complications have been described, including malunion, non-union, infection, avascular necrosis, heterotopic ossification, stiffness, and partial or complete growth arrest in children. Many of these complications may be related to the extensile surgical approaches sometimes necessary in addressing these injuries. We have begun using arthroscopic techniques in specific fracture patterns in an attempt to decrease some of these complications. In the hands of a skilled arthroscopist, these techniques can provide excellent visualization and enable anatomic repair of some intraarticular elbow fractures with minimal surgical dissection. Arthroscopy also allows for the preservation of soft tissue attachments. Improved instrumentation and surgical technique has expanded the indications for arthroscopy in soft tissue and bony repair in elbow trauma. Our preliminary data is encouraging, however, long-term studies and larger series are necessary.

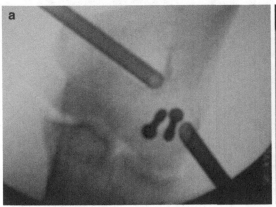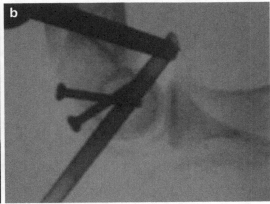

Fig. 11.14   Placement of cannulated screws for fixation of the fragment. (**a**) AP view. (**b**) Lateral view

References

1. Doornberg JN, Ring D. Coronoid fracture patterns. J Hand Surg Am 2006;31:45–52
2. Sanchez-Sotelo J, O'Driscoll SW, Morrey BF. Medial oblique compression fracture of the coronoid process of the ulna. J Shoulder Elbow Surg 2005;14:60–64
3. Pugh DM, Wild LM, Schemitsch EH, King GJ, McKee MD. Standard surgical protocol to treat elbow dislocations with radial head and coronoid fractures. J Bone Joint Surg Am 2004;86:1122–1130
4. Cage DJ, Abrams RA, Callahan JJ, Botte MJ. Soft tissue attachments of the ulnar coronoid process. An anatomic study with radiographic correlation. Clin Orthop Relat Res 1995 Nov; (320):154–158
5. Closky RF, Goode JR, Kirschenbaum D, Cody RP. The role of the coronoid process in elbow instability. A biomechanical analysis of axial loading. J Bone Joint Surg Am 2000;82:1749–1755
6. O'Driscoll SW, Bell DF, Morrey BF. Posterolateral rotatory instability of the elbow. J Bone Joint Surg Am 1991;73:440–446
7. O'Driscoll SW, Jupiter JB, Cohen MS, Ring D, McKee MD. Difficult elbow fractures: pearls and pitfalls. Instr Course Lect 2003;52:113–134
8. Regan W, Morrey BF. Fractures of the coronoid process of the ulna. J Bone Joint Surg Am 1989;71:1348–1354
9. Broberg MA, Morrey BF. Results of treatment of fracture-dislocations of the elbow. Clin Orthop Relat Res 1987 Mar;(216):109–19
10. Ring D, Jupiter JB, Simpson NS. Monteggia fractures in adults. J Bone Joint Surg Am 1998 Dec;80(12):1733–44
11. Lichtenburg R. A study of 2532 fractures in children. Am J Surg 1954;87:330–338
12. Flynn JC, Richards JF, Saltzman RI. Prevention and treatment of nonunion of slightly displaced fractures of the lateral humeral condyle in children. An end-result study. J Bone Joint Surg Am 1975;57:1087–1092
13. Milch H. Fractures and fracture-dislocations of humeral condyles. J Trauma 1964;4:592–607
14. Salter R, Harris W. Injuries involving the epiphyseal plate. J Bone Joint Surg Am 1963;45:587–592
15. Micheli LJ, Luke AC, Mintzer CM, et al. Elbow arthroscopy in the pediatric and adolescent population. Arthroscopy 2001;17(7):694–699
16. Dunn AL, Busch MT, Wyly JB, et al. Arthroscopic synovectomy for hemophilic joint disease in a pediatric population. J Pediatr Orthop 2004;24(4):414–426
17. Haraldsson S. On osteochondrosis deformas juvenilis capituli humeri including investigation of intraosseous vasculature in distal humerus. Acta Orthop Scand Suppl. 1959;38:1–23
18. Jakob R, Fowles JV, Rang M, et al. Observations concerning fractures of the lateral humeral condyle in children. J Bone Joint Surg Br 1975;57:430–436
19. Bernstein SM, King JD, Sanderson RA. Fractures of the medial epicondyle of the humerus. Contemp Orthop 1981;12:637–641
20. Skak SV, Olsen SD, Smaabrekke A. Deformity after fracture of the lateral humeral condyle in children. J Pediatr Orthop B 2001;10(2):142–152

Minimally Invasive Approaches for Lateral Epicondylitis

12

Bradford O. Parsons and Michael R. Hausman

Lateral epicondylitis is a painful condition that affects the lateral aspect of the elbow, usually centered around the epicondyle of the humerus. Historically called tennis elbow, this condition occurs in both men and women, usually in the 35- to 50-year age range, and rarely in tennis players. Patients present with laterally based elbow pain, exacerbated with repetitive stresses to the wrist and finger extensors, specifically the extensor carpi radialis brevis (ECRB) and extensor digitorum communis (EDC). A distinct pathoetiology has not been elucidated, and as such most patients have an idiopathic source, although some patients report "work-related" causes. Direct trauma is rarely a source of tennis elbow pain, neither is tennis, as only 5–10% of patients with lateral epicondylitis are tennis players [1]. Most patients report an insidious onset with pain associated with gripping, carrying, and holding objects with the forearm in pronation and the elbow in extension.

The natural history of tennis elbow is that it will usually resolve over time, but often with a protracted course. Numerous nonoperative and operative modalities to treat lateral epicondylitis have been described in the literature, although determining the "best" treatment is difficult if not impossible based on the literature [1–15]. Currently, most patients who are indicated for operative treatment of their painful tennis elbow are managed with one of two procedures, a formal open release, as described originally by Hohmann, and modified by Nirschl, or an arthroscopic release [6, 9]. A review of the literature will reveal support for both open and arthroscopic techniques, and until a well-designed prospective, randomized trial comparing these techniques is available, many surgeons are guided by "their subjective viewpoint and clinical experience." [16] As such, we will describe the open and the arthroscopic procedures to treat patients with tennis elbow, both of which adhere to the principles of minimally invasive procedures.

Pathoanatomy

Lateral epicondylitis pain is located near the origin of the extensor muscles at the lateral epicondyle, most frequently at the origin of the ECRB and EDC. The ECRB originates on the anterior aspect of the lateral epicondyle, deep to the EDC and inferior to the extensor carpi radialis longus (ECRL), which originates proximally on the flare of the lateral column just above the lateral epicondyle. The ECRL muscle is the most superficial and proximal muscle observed during tennis elbow open surgery, and serves as a guide to the ECRB, which is deep and distal to the muscle.

Although the ECRB has historically been implicated in lateral epicondylitis, anatomically there is no distinct division between the ECRB and EDC origins. Often, the pathologic lesion is

B.O. Parsons (✉)
Department of Orthopaedics, Mount Sinai School
of Medicine, New York, NY, USA
e-mail: bradford.parsons@mountsinai.org

observed in this confluent area. Additionally, the tendinous origins of the EDC and ECRB are confluent with the lateral ulnar collateral ligament (LUCL), which may be palpable as a stout band deep to the muscle [17]. Iatrogenic LUCL injuries following tennis elbow procedures have been reported and an understanding of the normal ligamentous anatomy of the lateral elbow is critical to preventing ligament injury and elbow instability [18, 19]. The LUCL originates off of the lateral epicondyle and inserts on the proximal ulna. The lesion associated with lateral epicondylitis is usually anterior to the LUCL and can be treated without damaging this critical structure.

Although often misrepresented as an inflammatory process, lateral epicondylitis does not involved acute inflammation. Biopsy specimen analyses of the pathologic tissue found at the ECRB and EDC origin have not shown acute or chronic inflammation, but have shown vascular proliferation, hyaline degeneration, and granulation tissue [2, 8, 15, 20–23]. Some have hypothesized that the changes seen on specimen analysis may be a result of some of the nonoperative treatments of lateral epicondylitis, such as cortisone injections [16].

Degeneration of the ECRB/EDC origin may not be the sole etiology of symptoms in patients who are diagnosed with lateral epicondylitis. Recently, one of us [8] described a meniscal-like fold of tissue that extends off of the radiocapitellar capsule and impinges on the radial head or interposes in the radiocapitellar joint in patients with symptoms of lateral epicondylitis, similar to a "snapping plica" lesion described by others (Fig. 12.1) [2, 24, 25]. This capsulosynovial fringe of tissue was found in a large subset of patients, and a cadaveric study also identified this same tissue in many specimens. In their series, the authors resected the pathologic fringe of tissue back to the native annular ligament. Subsequent to surgery, 28 of 30 patients subjectively graded their outcome as either better (4 patients) or much better (24 patients). The exact role this tissue has in patients with lateral epicondylitis remains to be seen, but an open technique often does not allow the identification of such pathologic lesions.

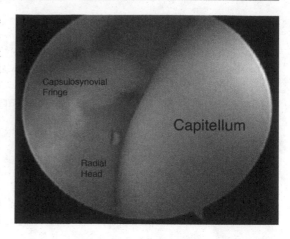

Fig. 12.1 Capsulosynovial fringe of tissue seen arthroscopically in many patients with lateral epicondylitis. Often this tissue can be found to be impinging on the radial head articular cartilage, causing synovitis and pain

Diagnosing Lateral Epicondylitis

Lateral epicondylitis is diagnosed by a careful history and physical examination. Patients often report a specific *event* that heralds the onset of their symptoms, but often, upon further investigation, an insidious onset is appreciated. As mentioned previously, rarely are patients tennis players. History should identify exacerbating activities, such as carrying objects with the wrist extended and the forearm pronated. Painful symptoms with gripping activities, such as turning a doorknob or holding objects (even as small as a toothbrush), should be elicited.

Mechanical symptoms, such as locking or clicking, may describe an intraarticular source, such as loose bodies, or a capsulosynovial fold. Additionally, any symptoms of instability, especially in the face of failed open tennis elbow surgery, should be elicited. Often, these patients will describe vague pain with activities that mimic the lateral pivot shift maneuver, such as rising out of an armchair by pushing off with the triceps. Patients who report numbness or tingling or shooting pains often have a neurologic source of their pain, such as radial tunnel. Often the subtle differences in radial tunnel and tennis elbow can be identified by physical examination.

Patients with tennis elbow have tenderness at the ECRB/EDC origin, often one fingerbreadth distal and anterior to the tip of the lateral epicondyle. Pain is exacerbated with provocative maneuvers. These include pain with resisted wrist extension, more so with the elbow in extension versus flexion. Pain can also be elicited with resisted long finger extension. Gripping with the elbow in extension can also evoke painful symptoms. Often, symptoms are less dramatic with these provocative maneuvers performed in elbow flexion versus elbow extension, especially gripping tests.

Clicking over the radiocapitellar joint while moving the elbow through an arc of motion, or tenderness over the joint line, may indicate an intraarticular source, such as loose bodies or a plica. A provocative test for a symptomatic plica can be performed by moving the elbow through an arc of motion while the patient holds their forearm in pronation and wrist in resisted extension [24]. This maneuver causes a large plica to "snap" back and forth into the radiocapitellar joint.

Patients with lateral epicondylitis need to be differentiated from those with radial tunnel syndrome. Radial tunnel syndrome is caused by compression of the posterior interosseous nerve in the radial tunnel. These patients often have more poorly localized pain, often distal to the epicondyle, and may also have wrist aching or complaints of "heaviness" in the forearm or wrist. Tenderness is elicited in the area of the radial tunnel, not over the ECRB/EDC origin. Pain may be exacerbated by resisted supination or resisted long finger extension. It is possible for patients to have findings of both lateral epicondylitis and radial tunnel, and differentiating the primary problem may be difficult. An injection of local anesthetic, with or without cortisone, can be helpful in determining the exact source of symptoms.

Plain radiograph results of the elbow are often normal in patients with lateral epicondylitis, but may reveal a degenerative changes or loose bodies. Magnetic resonance imaging (MRI) is used in patients whose diagnosis is not obvious, or in those patients where suspicion that an intraarticular lesion, such as a plica, may be present. However, the utility of MRI in evaluation of these patients has not been validated, and is often not necessary. Electromyogram (EMG) analysis is not usually helpful in diagnosing radial tunnel syndrome, which remains a diagnosis based on the history and physical examination.

Nonoperative Management

Most patients with symptoms of lateral epicondylitis will improve with nonoperative measures and time, although a long course is often observed. Numerous nonoperative modalities have been attempted, with little validation of their success, including bracing, acupuncture, ultrasound, extracorporeal shock wave therapy, and laser treatment, among many others [4, 5, 7, 12, 14]. We find that a mainstay of nonoperative management is patient education and activity modification in an effort to diminish inciting or exacerbating activities. Patients should learn to carry objects with the forearm supinated and wrist straight. Avoiding grip or wrist extension often is helpful in alleviating symptoms. Laborers who perform repetitive activities, especially those requiring substantial force across the extensor origin, should have duties restricted and modified. Additionally, the use of tools that generate vibratory forces should be restricted.

Patients may benefit from a home-based physical therapy regimen aimed at stretching and strengthening the extensors, while using modalities such as ice and heat to reduce pain and improve mobility. Additionally, counterforce braces are often used to relieve pressure on the ECRB origin, thereby (in theory) allowing the body to heal the degenerative tissue. Finally, patients with acute painful processes may get symptomatic relief from a steroid injection, although most series report temporary relief in patients, often those previously untreated for their symptoms [11, 26].

Surgical Indications

While some [21] have outlined specific indications for surgical management of patients with tennis elbow, many patients "fail" nonoperative measures because of the impact symptoms have on their ability to work or their quality of life. Such patients, especially if temporary relief was obtained with a steroid injection, are candidates for operative treatment. All patients are initially managed nonoperatively with a rehabilitation program and steroid injection, and those patients whose symptoms do not improve enough or within an acceptable modicum of time are offered surgery.

Determining which surgery to perform for patients with lateral epicondylitis can be more difficult then choosing which patients should be indicated. No consensus of procedure, whether percutaneous, open, or arthroscopic can be clearly gleaned from the current literature. Nearly all procedures currently utilize mini-incisions and avoid extensive exposures. Therefore, we describe both the traditional open approach as well as the arthroscopic procedure we use.

Patients who have classic signs and symptoms of lateral epicondylitis are amenable to an open release, as are those with recurrent symptoms. Additionally, any patients with symptoms of posterolateral rotatory instability will require open surgery, as ligament reconstruction is likely to be required. Conversely, those with signs and symptoms of intraarticular lesions, such as mechanical symptoms, are indicated for arthroscopic management. In our practice, we have transitioned to performing nearly all tennis elbow procedures arthroscopically because of the ability to evaluate the joint and look for synovial folds and plicas, as well as debride the ECRB origin (if pathologic).

Contraindications

There are no specific contraindications for surgical management of patients with lateral epicondylitis. Most errors of management come following inaccurate diagnosis or failure to appreciate subtle instability or joint derangement. Obviously, patients who are unable to undergo anesthesia are not candidates, and are managed nonoperatively.

Surgical Procedure: Open Lateral Epicondylitis Debridement

Patient Positioning

Patients are positioned supine with the arm on a hand table. Either regional or general anesthesia can be used. A tourniquet is placed on the upper arm, and the extremity is draped free distal to the tourniquet. The hand is covered with a stockinet.

Procedure

Once the patient is anesthetized and draped, the incision is marked out. The lateral epicondyle and radiocapitellar joint is identified and marked, and the incision is marked along a line from the epicondyle toward Lister's tubercle distally, measuring 2–3 cm (Fig. 12.2). The arm is exsanguinated and the tourniquet is inflated to 100 mmHg above systolic blood pressure. The incision is carried down to the fascia of the extensor muscles. Identification of the ECRL fascia is the landmark to finding the ECRB. The thin fascia with muscle tissue present is the ECRL, while the thicker fascia posteriorly represents the EDC. The ECRB fascia will be deep and anterior to the ECRL fascia.

At this point, the fascial septae are palpated to discern the orientation of the LUCL, which divides the radiocapitellar joint into two hemispheres. The LUCL will feel as a thickened band of the fascia. The fascia of the ECRL is then incised just anterior to the LUCL, along the length of the skin incision. The ECRB/EDC origins are now exposed. Often at this point, the degenerated, pathologic tissue of lateral epicondylitis can be identified in the origin (Fig. 12.3). The pathologic tissue is excised sharply starting distally at the boundary of pathologic and normal tissue, extending proximally to the origin off of the lateral epicondyle. Often the entire thickness of the portion of the ECRB/EDC involved is removed, although care should be taken to not violate the joint capsule at this point.

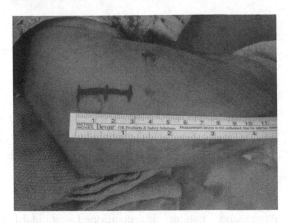

Fig. 12.2 Skin incision for open tennis elbow release. The incision is along a line from the anterior aspect of the lateral epicondyle to Lister's tubercle in the wrist. Usually, a few centimeters are sufficient

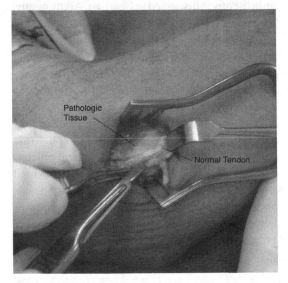

Fig. 12.3 Pathologic tissue often observed during open tennis elbow release

The anterior limit of dissection is the muscle of the ECRL, while posteriorly it is the normal portion of the EDC tendinous origin. Some authors have advocated burring or drilling the bone of the lateral epicondyle after all pathologic tissue has been removed [3, 9, 21]. In theory this helps bring fresh blood into the area and help healing, but we have found, as have others [27, 28], that this increases perioperative pain and may delay recovery. Therefore, we do not decorticate the lateral epicondyle at the origin of the ECRB.

Patients with suspected intraarticular pathology should have the joint inspected through a small capsulotomy, although exposure is limited through this mini-incision approach, and therefore an arthroscopic evaluation may be more appropriate. To expose the joint, the anterolateral capsule of the radiocapitellar joint is incised from the anterior column distally. Utmost care should be taken to not violate the LUCL, which originates on the epicondyle. By incising the anterolateral capsule of the radiocapitellar joint, the capsulotomy will remain in the anterior hemisphere of the joint and should not violate the LUCL. The supinator muscle fibers are often encountered distally over the radiocapitellar joint and can be bluntly dissected off of the capsule and retracted to give a little more distal exposure. This will allow limited exposure of the radiocapitellar joint.

The wound is then irrigated with normal saline and the joint capsule (if opened) is closed with 3–0 Vicryl suture. The anterior and posterior fascial edges are then approximated together with a 2–0 Vicryl suture. We do not repair the fascia back to the epicondyle through bone tunnels or using suture anchors, but rather repair the fascia together in a side-to-side method. The skin is repaired using a 3–0 Monocryl suture in the dermis and a 4–0 running subcuticular stitch. The wound is dressed with Steri-Strips and a bandage. The elbow is initially immobilized in a long arm splint in 90° flexion and the wrist in slight dorsiflexion.

Rehabilitation

The splint is removed at the first postoperative visit at 7–10 days, and active range of motion exercises of the elbow, wrist, and hand are started. Additionally, the patient is allowed to use the extremity for activities of daily living. A removable wrist splint with dorsiflexion cock-up is given for comfort if needed. Strengthening exercises are begun at 6 weeks with unrestricted use of the extremity beginning at 3 months.

Surgical Technique: Arthroscopic Lateral Epicondylitis Release

Patient Positioning

Either regional or general anesthesia may be used. Arthroscopic release may be performed in either the lateral decubitus or supine position, as preferred by the surgeon. The lateral decubitus positioning will be described here. The patient is positioned lateral decubitus on a beanbag with care to pad the all bony prominences and ensure no pressure is placed on the peroneal nerve of the contralateral leg. A tourniquet is placed around the upper arm and the extremity is draped free with a stockinet placed over the hand. The extremity is placed over a lateral elbow positioner so that the arm is parallel to the floor, and the elbow flexed 90°. The arm is positioned so that the holder is at the midpoint of the humerus, just distal to the tourniquet. Care should be taken to ensure further flexion is possible without impingement of the hand against the operating table, and that instruments can be utilized without impingement against the holder prior to draping.

Instrumentation

Standard arthroscopic instruments are used, including a 4.0-mm, 30° arthroscope and 5.5-mm unfenestrated cannulas. A full radius 3.5-mm shaver is used, as is an electrocautery ablation device. Extra switching sticks (preferably pointed, not blunt tip) are used to retract during arthroscopy. A spinal needle is used to localize portal placement from an inside-out technique. Occasionally a banana blade is also used to remove a capsulosynovial fringe when present.

Procedure

After the patient is positioned, standard arthroscopic portals are marked, including a proximal anteromedial, an anterolateral, a transtriceps posterior, and a posterolateral portal (a detailed discussion of portal placement in elbow arthroscopy is discussed in Chap. 8). Additionally, the palpable landmarks are also marked, including the medial epicondyle, medial intermuscular septum, capitellum, radial head, and the course of the ulnar nerve (Fig. 12.4). The arm is then exsanguinated and the tourniquet raised to 100 mmHg over systolic pressure.

The joint is then insufflated with 25 cc of normal saline via the direct lateral "soft spot" (the center of a triangle formed by the lateral epicondyle, radial head, and olecranon). The proximal anteromedial portal is incised and bluntly developed with a clamp, taking care to remain anterior to the intermuscular septum. The 4.0-mm trochar and camera sleeve are then placed into the joint

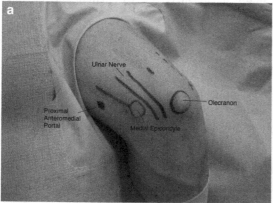
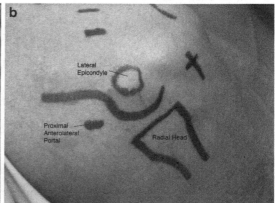

Fig. 12.4 Position and surface landmarks for arthroscopic tennis elbow release. (**a**) The medial landmarks include the medial epicondyle (*circle*), ulnar nerve, and medial intramuscular septum (*line*). (**b**) Laterally, the epicondyle (*circle*), radial head, and capitellum are landmarks. Standard portals are marked

just above the trochlea, with joint penetration confirmed by backflow of fluid through the cannula outflow.

The 4.0-mm, 30° arthroscopic camera is then introduced and a diagnostic arthroscopy is performed of the anterior joint. Under direct visualization, the working anterolateral portal is made by introducing a spinal needle into the joint so that it enters just anterior to the junction of the capitellum and lateral column, at the ECRB-capsular attachment to the lateral column. The portal should be made proximal enough to allow an angle of approach to the anterior capsular tissue of the radiocapitellar joint. Once established, a smooth cannula is introduced over a pointed switching stick into the lateral portal. The 3.5-mm shaver is then used through the lateral working portal to debride any synovitis and clean the anterolateral capsule.

Often a capsulosynovial fold will be observed adherent to the annular ligament and radial head, occasionally interposing into the radiocapitellar joint (Fig. 12.1). When observed, this tissue is removed to expose the native annular ligament and uncover the radial head. It has been one of our experiences that this often seems to be the source of pain in these patients. The aberrant capsular tissue is removed using a combination of shaver, electrocautery ablation, and occasionally a banana blade for tough, resistant tissue. Care is taken to protect the radial head articular cartilage, which, once exposed, often reveals areas of contact degeneration as a result of direct pressure from the pathologic capsular folds (Fig. 12.5).

After removal of this tissue, attention is then turned to the anterolateral capsule and overlying ECRB/EDC origin. Often this area is synovitic in patients with tennis elbow. The capsule is removed with electrocautery, starting proximally at the junction of the anterior capitellum and lateral column. The capsule is removed from deep to superficial, at which point the tendon of the ECRB and EDC is visible. The capsule is removed distally to the level of the radiocapitellar joint, taking care to remain in the anterior hemisphere of the capitellum to protect the LUCL. Once the capsule is removed, the ECRB/EDC tendon origins are removed with the shaver until healthy muscle fibers (ECRL) are exposed.

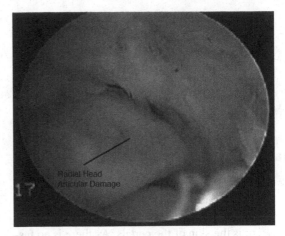

Fig. 12.5 Damaged radial head articular cartilage observed after resection of impinging capsulosynovial fringe of pathologic tissue during elbow arthroscopy

Often, patients with intraarticular-based symptoms or synovitis anteriorly will have posterior or posterolateral compartment involvement as well. The posterior transtriceps portal is developed, along with a proximal posterolateral (working) portal to evaluate the posterior compartment of the elbow. The olecranon and olecranon fossa are evaluated, and if normal attention is taken, to the posterolateral gutter, especially in patients who had the aforementioned pathologic capsulosynovial fold compressing the radiocapitellar joint. This tissue frequently extends posterolaterally to encroach on the radial head and radiocapitellar joint, and if the posterolateral gutter is not visualized, this tissue will be missed.

The posterolateral gutter is entered by placing the arthroscope in the proximal posterolateral (working) portal, and passing it posterior to the capitellum, just lateral to the olecranon. Once confirmation of location is obtained by visualizing the radial head and sigmoid notch of the ulna, a distal posterolateral (accessory or radiocapitellar) portal is made under direct visualization. Any synovitis or pathologic capsular tissue is removed by shaving and electrocautery. Care is taken to not violate the LUCL, which travels along the lateral aspect of the joint, from the epicondyle around the radial head onto the ulna. By working more medially along the lateral surface of the ulna and around the radial head, the LUCL can be avoided.

After all debridement is completed, the joint is copiously irrigated with fluid and the portals are closed with interrupted nylon stitches, with care taken to obtain a watertight closure in an effort to prevent sinus formation. The wounds are dressed and the elbow is placed in a posterior splint for immobilization.

Rehabilitation

One of the advantages of an arthroscopic debridement is that the only "healing" that needs to occur is the skin of the portals. As there is no fascial repair, the elbow does not need to be protected. As such, the splint and bandages are removed after 3 days by the patient, and the patient is allowed to use the elbow for activities of daily living within their limits of discomfort. Stitches are removed at the first postoperative visit in 7–10 days. As perioperative pain resolves, the patient is allowed to resume all activities, including athletics. Formal rehabilitation is reserved for the rare patient who develops perioperative stiffness of the elbow.

Results

Many patients with tennis elbow improve with time and nonoperative measures, however, patients with recalcitrant symptoms often undergo surgical treatment. The surgical management of lateral epicondylitis has been the source of much debate, with multiple procedures described, most with similar results. Most series report 80–85% of patients obtaining "good to excellent" results, with few prospective series available for analysis [3, 6, 8–10, 15, 16, 21, 27–30]. Hohmann reported 86–88% satisfactory results following the original description of open release of patients with tennis elbow in 1933 [6]. Nirschl and Pettrone cited 85% good to excellent results in their review of 88 elbows treated with their modified open release, which included isolated debridement of the pathologic tendon tissue, decortication of the epicondyle, and repair of the ECRL [9]. Additionally, 85% of their patients returned to full activity, including sports. Subsequently, the

Nirschl technique became the "gold standard" in the surgical management of patients with tennis elbow.

Similar reports are found with more recent analyses of open procedures. Zingg and Schneeberger reported 81% of 21 patients had a satisfactory outcome with no or mild pain [28]. However, they voiced concern over the prolonged perioperative recovery following open release using the modified Nirschl method. They found similar results to Khashaba, who reported increased pain and greater stiffness in patients who had decortication and drilling of the epicondyle compared with those who had just release in a prospective, randomized series of 23 elbows [27]. Based on these recent investigations, we currently debride the pathologic tissue during open release, but do not decorticate or drill the epicondyle.

Concerns over perioperative pain and delayed recovery following open repair, as well as allowing for an intraarticular evaluation, led many surgeons to perform arthroscopic releases of the ECRB/EDC origin to manage tennis elbow [8, 10, 29, 30]. Peart et al. found that 72% of arthroscopic releases had good to excellent outcomes, similar to the 69% following open release, but the patients treated arthroscopically recovered and returned to work faster [10]. Stapleton and Baker reported faster recovery and quicker return to sports in a review of open versus arthroscopically treated elbows (35 vs. 66 days for return to sport) [30]. They also found that 60% of patients treated arthroscopically had associated intraarticular disorders. A later study by Kaminsky and Baker reported that 95% of 39 patients were "better" or "much better" following arthroscopic release [29]. Similarly, in a series performed at our institution, Mullet et al. reported 93% of 39 patients were "better" or "much better" following arthroscopic debridement. The patients in this series returned to work at an average of 7 days [8].

We have found arthroscopic release allows for the potential of quicker recovery, often resulting in less need for rehabilitation. Additionally, associated intraarticular lesions, especially any capsulo-synovial folds impinging on the radiocapitellar joint, can be removed, whereas they may be missed following an open release. Although having many potential advantages, elbow arthroscopy is technically challenging and has a substantial learning curve, and is not without complication, such as nerve injury. As such, until a prospective, randomized trial examining arthroscopic versus open release is performed, a clear answer as to the "gold standard" approach will be lacking.

Conclusion

Most patients with lateral epicondylitis will obtain symptomatic improvement with nonoperative modalities. Occasionally, however, patients cannot tolerate their symptoms, or are not improving expeditiously enough and can benefit from surgical intervention. As with many other areas of orthopedic surgery, a trend toward minimally invasive surgical techniques has occurred, and the treatment of tennis elbow is no different. Traditional open techniques involve minimally dissection and exposure, and with more surgeons becoming comfortable with arthroscopic elbow surgery, the surgical management of tennis elbow has become truly minimally invasive. Arthroscopy offers many advantages, including visualization of the entire joint, faster recovery (including return to work), and results compare favorably to many of the reports of traditional open techniques.

References

1. Assendelft WJ, Hay EM, Adshead R, Bouter LM. Corticosteroid injections for lateral epicondylitis: a systematic overview. Br J Gen Pract 1996;46(405): 209–216
2. Bosworth DM. The role of the orbicular ligament in tennis elbow. J Bone Joint Surg Am 1955;37-A(3): 527–533
3. Dunkow PD, Jatti M, Muddu BN. A comparison of open and percutaneous techniques in the surgical treatment of tennis elbow. J Bone Joint Surg Br 2004;86(5):701–704
4. Haker E, Lundeberg T. Pulsed ultrasound treatment in lateral epicondylalgia. Scand J Rehabil Med 1991; 23(3):115–118
5. Harding W. Use and misuse of the tennis elbow strap. Phys Sportsmed 1992;20:65–74
6. Hohmann G. Das Wesen und die Behandlung des sogenannten Tennisellbogens. Munch Med Wochesnschr 1933;80:250–252
7. Molsberger A, Hille E. The analgesic effect of acupuncture in chronic tennis elbow pain. Br J Rheumatol 1994;33(12):1162–1165
8. Mullett H, Sprague M, Brown G, Hausman M. Arthroscopic treatment of lateral epicondylitis: clinical and cadaveric studies. Clin Orthop Relat Res 2005;439:123–128
9. Nirschl RP, Pettrone FA. Tennis elbow. The surgical treatment of lateral epicondylitis. J Bone Joint Surg Am 1979;61(6A):832–839
10. Peart RE, Strickler SS, Schweitzer KM, Jr. Lateral epicondylitis: a comparative study of open and arthroscopic lateral release. Am J Orthop 2004;33(11): 565–567
11. Price R, Sinclair H, Heinrich I, Gibson T. Local injection treatment of tennis elbow - hydrocortisone, triamcinolone and lignocaine compared. Br J Rheumatol 1991;30(1):39–44
12. Rompe JD, Hopf C, Kullmer K, Heine J, Burger R, Nafe B. Low-energy extracorporal shock wave therapy for persistent tennis elbow. Int Orthop 1996;20(1): 23–27
13. Smidt N, van der Windt DA, Assendelft WJ, Deville WL, Korthals-de Bos IB, Bouter LM. Corticosteroid injections, physiotherapy, or a wait-and-see policy for lateral epicondylitis: a randomised controlled trial. Lancet 2002;359(9307):657–662
14. Vasseljen O, Jr, Hoeg N, Kjeldstad B, Johnsson A, Larsen S. Low level laser versus placebo in the treatment of tennis elbow. Scand J Rehabil Med 1992;24(1): 37–42
15. Verhaar J, Walenkamp G, Kester A, van Mameren H, van der Linden T. Lateral extensor release for tennis elbow. A prospective long-term follow-up study. J Bone Joint Surg Am 1993;75(7):1034–1043
16. Boyer MI, Hastings H, II. Lateral tennis elbow: "Is there any science out there?" J Shoulder Elbow Surg 1999;8(5):481–491
17. Cohen MS, Hastings H, II. Rotatory instability of the elbow. The anatomy and role of the lateral stabilizers. J Bone Joint Surg Am 1997;79(2):225–233
18. Kalainov DM, Cohen MS. Posterolateral rotatory instability of the elbow in association with lateral epicondylitis. A report of three cases. J Bone Joint Surg Am 2005;87(5):1120–1125
19. Morrey BF. Reoperation for failed treatment of refractory lateral epicondylitis. J Shoulder Elbow Surg 1992;1:47–55
20. Bosworth DM. Surgical treatment of tennis elbow; a follow-up study. J Bone Joint Surg Am 1965;47(8): 1533–1536
21. Nirschl RP. Elbow tendinosis/tennis elbow. Clin Sports Med 1992;11(4):851–870
22. Potter HG, Hannafin JA, Morwessel RM, DiCarlo EF, O'Brien SJ, Altchek DW. Lateral epicondylitis: correlation of MR imaging, surgical, and histopathologic findings. Radiology 1995;196(1):43–46

23. Regan W, Wold LE, Coonrad R, Morrey BF. Microscopic histopathology of chronic refractory lateral epicondylitis. Am J Sports Med 1992;20(6): 746–749

24. Antuna SA, O'Driscoll SW. Snapping plicae associated with radiocapitellar chondromalacia. Arthroscopy 2001;17(5):491–495

25. Duparc F, Putz R, Michot C, Muller JM, Freger P. The synovial fold of the humeroradial joint: anatomical and histological features, and clinical relevance in lateral epicondylalgia of the elbow. Surg Radiol Anat 2002;24(5):302–307

26. Solveborn SA, Buch F, Mallmin H, Adalberth G. Cortisone injection with anesthetic additives for radial epicondylalgia (tennis elbow). Clin Orthop Relat Res 1995;(316):99–105

27. Khashaba A. Nirschl tennis elbow release with or without drilling. Br J Sports Med 2001;35(3): 200–201

28. Zingg PO, Schneeberger AG. Debridement of extensors and drilling of the lateral epicondyle for tennis elbow: a retrospective follow-up study. J Shoulder Elbow Surg 2006;15(3):347–350

29. Kaminsky SB, Baker CL, Jr. Lateral epicondylitis of the elbow. Tech Hand Up Extrem Surg 2003;7(4):179–189

30. Stapleton TR, Baker, CL. Arthroscopic treatment of lateral epicondylitis: a clinical study [abstract]. Arthroscopy 1996;12:365–366

Overview of Wrist and Hand Approaches: Indications for Minimally Invasive Techniques

13

Steve K. Lee

Orthopedic surgery has seen a recent explosion of minimally invasive techniques [1–7] and the wrist and hand are no exception. These techniques range from percutaneous, endoscopic, arthroscopic, to mini-open procedures. The main topics covered in the following chapters include minimally invasive fixation for wrist fractures, endoscopic carpal tunnel release, minimally invasive trigger finger release, and minimally invasive treatment of finger fractures. Indications and advantages of minimally invasive wrist and hand surgery will be discussed as well as detailed descriptions of these new surgical techniques.

Similar to advantages proposed in other regions of orthopedic surgery, the advantages of minimally invasive techniques for surgery of the wrist and hand include shorter recovery times, earlier return to work, and less scar tissue formation with potentially improved outcomes [8, 9]. Advances in visualization via endoscopic and arthroscopic cameras and improved anatomic knowledge for increased safety during minimally invasive approaches have helped expand the use and experience in these techniques.

S.K. Lee (✉)
Division of Hand Surgery, Department
of Orthopaedic Surgery, The NYU Hospital
for Joint Diseases, New York, NY, USA

Department of Orthopaedic Surgery, The New York
University School of Medicine, New York, NY, USA

Hand Surgery Service,
Bellevue Hospital Center, New York, NY, USA
e-mail: steve.lee@nyumc.org

Regarding wrist fractures, the surgeon has a wide range of options for distal radius fracture operative treatment, such as external fixation, open reduction and internal fixation with fixed-angle plates and other devices, and minimally invasive techniques of percutaneous intrafocal Kapandji pinning, mini-open reduction and bone grafting, and arthroscopic reduction and fixation, among others [10–16]. Distal to the radial platform, the main paradigm for minimally invasive carpal bone fracture treatment is arthroscopic reduction and internal fixation of scaphoid fractures championed by Slade and others [17–21].

Endoscopic carpal tunnel release has been shown to decrease recovery times with earlier return to work [8, 9]. Generally, outcomes are similar to open carpal tunnel release after 3 months [22]. Potential complications range from failure of surgery from incomplete release to reversible and irreversible nerve injury [23–27]. There are two major types of endoscopic carpal tunnel release: the one-incision technique of Agee [28], and the two-incision technique of Chow [29, 30].

Trigger finger release has classically been performed with an open technique of a 1- to 2-cm incision, either transversely, obliquely, or longitudinally placed. Minimally invasive techniques include percutaneous with a hypodermic needle, endoscopic, and mini-open with special trigger digit devices [31–40].

Regarding hand fractures, it is generally accepted that the less dissection and open exposure is performed, the better the results. Open approaches run the risk of increased scarring between bone and the soft tissues of tendon, ligament, and skin. When possible, closed reduction and internal fixation (usually by percutaneous pinning) is preferable [41–44]. Percutaneous pinning minimizes scarring, the hardware is inexpensive and readily available, and the hardware is easy to remove in the office. Recent new reduction clamps with built-in pin guides help simplify the pinning.

External fixation and other minimally invasive techniques have been described [45–48]. Arthroscopic reduction and internal fixation has been described for intraarticular fractures of the metacarpophalangeal joints of the thumb and fingers [50], the carpometacarpal joint of the thumb (basal joint), and the proximal interphalangeal joints of the fingers. Small joint arthroscopy is a relatively new technique and does not enjoy as widespread use as its larger cousins. Continued advances in miniature optics and surgical techniques will spawn new advances in minimally invasive treatment techniques of hand fractures.

The following chapters discuss in depth specific techniques of minimally invasive wrist and hand surgery. Special emphasis will be on indications, advantages of minimally invasive techniques, anatomy, surgical technique, and pearls and pitfalls.

References

1. Bottner F, Delgado S, Sculco TP. Minimally invasive total hip replacement: the posterolateral approach. American Journal of Orthopedics (Belle Mead, N.J.) 2006;35(5):218–24
2. Egol KA. Minimally invasive orthopaedic trauma surgery: a review of the latest techniques. Bulletin (Hospital for Joint Diseases (New York, N.Y.)) 2004; 62(1–2):6–12
3. Klein GR, Parvizi J, Sharkey PF, Rothman RH, Hozack WJ. Minimally invasive total hip arthroplasty: internet claims made by members of the Hip Society. Clinical Orthopaedics and Related Research 2005 Dec;(441):68–70
4. Langlotz K. Minimally invasive approaches in orthopaedic surgery. Minimally Invasive Therapy and Allied Technologies 2003;12(1):19–24
5. Lehman RA, Jr., Vaccaro AR, Bertagnoli R, Kuklo TR. Standard and minimally invasive approaches to the spine. The Orthopedic Clinics of North America 2005;36(3):281–92

6. Nogler M. Navigated minimal invasive total hip arthroplasty. Surgical Technology International 2004; 12:259–62
7. Wall EJ, Bylski-Austrow DI, Kolata RJ, Crawford AH. Endoscopic mechanical spinal hemiepiphysiodesis modifies spine growth. Spine 2005;30(10): 1148–53
8. Saw NL, Jones S, Shepstone L, Meyer M, Chapman PG, Logan AM. Early outcome and cost-effectiveness of endoscopic versus open carpal tunnel release: a randomized prospective trial. The Journal of Hand Surgery (Edinburgh, Lothian) 2003;28(5):444–9
9. Trumble TE, Diao E, Abrams RA, Gilbert-Anderson MM. Single-portal endoscopic carpal tunnel release compared with open release: a prospective, randomized trial. The Journal of Bone and Joint Surgery American 2002;84-A(7):1107–15
10. Weil WM, Trumble TE. Treatment of distal radius fractures with intrafocal (kapandji) pinning and supplemental skeletal stabilization. Hand Clinics 2005; 21(3):317–28
11. Duncan SF, Weiland AJ. Minimally invasive reduction and osteosynthesis of articular fractures of the distal radius. Injury 2001;32(Suppl 1): SA14–24
12. Ring D, Jupiter JB. Percutaneous and limited open fixation of fractures of the distal radius. Clinical Orthopaedics and Related Research 2000 Jun;(375): 105–15
13. Geissler WB, Fernandes D. Percutaneous and limited open reduction of intra-articular distal radial fractures. Hand Surgery 2000;5(2):85–92
14. Auge WK, II, Velazquez PA. The application of indirect reduction techniques in the distal radius: the role of adjuvant arthroscopy. Arthroscopy 2000;16(8): 830–5
15. Trumble TE, Wagner W, Hanel DP, Vedder NB, Gilbert M. Intrafocal (Kapandji) pinning of distal radius fractures with and without external fixation. The Journal of Hand Surgery 1998;23(3):381–94
16. Naidu SH, Capo JT, Moulton M, Ciccone W, II, Radin A. Percutaneous pinning of distal radius fractures: a biomechanical study. The Journal of Hand Surgery 1997;22(2):252–7
17. Slade JF, III, Grauer JN, Mahoney JD. Arthroscopic reduction and percutaneous fixation of scaphoid fractures with a novel dorsal technique. The Orthopedic Clinics of North America 2001;32(2):247–61
18. Slade JF, III, Jaskwhich D. Percutaneous fixation of scaphoid fractures. Hand Clinics 2001;17(4):553–74
19. Slade JF, III, Gutow AP, Geissler WB. Percutaneous internal fixation of scaphoid fractures via an arthroscopically assisted dorsal approach. The Journal of Bone and Joint Surgery American 2002;84-A(Suppl 2): 21–36
20. Slade JF, III, Geissler WB, Gutow AP, Merrell GA. Percutaneous internal fixation of selected scaphoid nonunions with an arthroscopically assisted dorsal approach. The Journal of Bone and Joint Surgery American 2003;85-A (Suppl 4):20–32

21. Slade JF, III, Dodds SD. Minimally invasive management of scaphoid nonunions. Clinical Orthopaedics and Related Research 2006 Apr;(445):108–19
22. Macdermid JC, Richards RS, Roth JH, Ross DC, King GJ. Endoscopic versus open carpal tunnel release: a randomized trial. The Journal of Hand Surgery 2003; 28(3):475–80
23. Thoma A, Veltri K, Haines T, Duku E. A meta-analysis of randomized controlled trials comparing endoscopic and open carpal tunnel decompression. Plastic and Reconstructive Surgery 2004;114(5):1137–46
24. Kretschmer T, Antoniadis G, Borm W, Richter HP. [Pitfalls of endoscopic carpal tunnel release]. Der Chirurg; Zeitschrift fur alle Gebiete der operativen Medizen 2004;75(12):1207–9
25. Thoma A, Veltri K, Haines T, Duku E. A systematic review of reviews comparing the effectiveness of endoscopic and open carpal tunnel decompression. Plastic and Reconstructive Surgery 2004;113(4):1184–91
26. Uchiyama S, Yasutomi T, Fukuzawa T, Nakagawa H, Kamimura M, Miyasaka T. Median nerve damage during two-portal endoscopic carpal tunnel release. Clinical Neurophysiology 2004;115(1):59–63
27. Varitimidis SE, Herndon JH, Sotereanos DG. Failed endoscopic carpal tunnel release. Operative findings and results of open revision surgery. The Journal of Hand Surgery (Edinburgh, Lothian) 1999;24(4):465–7
28. Agee JM, Peimer CA, Pyrek JD, Walsh WE. Endoscopic carpal tunnel release: a prospective study of complications and surgical experience. The Journal of Hand Surgery 1995;20(2):165–71; discussion 172
29. Chow JC, Hantes ME. Endoscopic carpal tunnel release: thirteen years' experience with the Chow technique. The Journal of Hand Surgery 2002;27(6): 1011–8
30. Chow JC. Endoscopic release of the carpal ligament for carpal tunnel syndrome: long-term results using the Chow technique. Arthroscopy 1999;15(4):417–21
31. Slesarenko YA, Mallo G, Hurst LC, Sampson SP, Serra-Hsu F. Percutaneous release of A1 pulley. Techniques in Hand & Upper Extremity Surgery 2006;10(1):54–6
32. Ragoowansi R, Acornley A, Khoo CT. Percutaneous trigger finger release: the "lift-cut" technique. British Journal of Plastic Surgery 2005;58(6):817–21
33. Wilhelmi BJ, Mowlavi A, Neumeister MW, Bueno R, Lee WP. Safe treatment of trigger finger with longitudinal and transverse landmarks: an anatomic study of the border fingers for percutaneous release. Plastic and Reconstructive Surgery 2003;112(4):993–9
34. Wilhelmi BJ, Snyder NT, Verbesey JE, Ganchi PA, Lee WP. Trigger finger release with hand surface

landmark ratios: an anatomic and clinical study. Plastic and Reconstructive Surgery 2001;108(4):908–15
35. Blumberg N, Arbel R, Dekel S. Percutaneous release of trigger digits. The Journal of Hand Surgery (Edinburgh, Lothian) 2001;26(3):256–7
36. Ha KI, Park MJ, Ha CW. Percutaneous release of trigger digits. The Journal of Bone and Joint Surgery 2001;83(1):75–7
37. Dunn MJ, Pess GM. Percutaneous trigger finger release: a comparison of a new push knife and a 19-gauge needle in a cadaveric model. The Journal of Hand Surgery 1999;24(4):860–5
38. Cihantimur B, Akin S, Ozcan M. Percutaneous treatment of trigger finger. 34 fingers followed 0.5–2 years. Acta Orthopaedica Scandinavica 1998;69(2):167–8
39. Bain GI, Turnbull J, Charles MN, Roth JH, Richards RS. Percutaneous A1 pulley release: a cadaveric study. The Journal of Hand Surgery 1995;20(5):781–4; discussion 785–6
40. Pope DF, Wolfe SW. Safety and efficacy of percutaneous trigger finger release. The Journal of Hand Surgery 1995;20(2):280–3
41. Geissler WB. Cannulated percutaneous fixation of intra-articular hand fractures. Hand Clinics 2006;22(3): 297–305, vi
42. Sawaizumi T, Nanno M, Nanbu A, Ito H. Percutaneous leverage pinning in the treatment of Bennett's fracture. Journal of Orthopaedic Science 2005;10(1): 27–31
43. Galanakis I, Aligizakis A, Katonis P, Papadokostakis G, Stergiopoulos K, Hadjipavlou A. Treatment of closed unstable metacarpal fractures using percutaneous transverse fixation with Kirschner wires. The Journal of Trauma 2003;55(3):509–13
44. Klein DM, Belsole RJ. Percutaneous treatment of carpal, metacarpal, and phalangeal injuries. Clinical Orthopaedics and Related Research 2000 Jun;(375): 116–25
45. Freeland AE, Orbay JL. Extraarticular hand fractures in adults: a review of new developments. Clinical Orthopaedics and Related Research 2006 Apr;(445): 133–45
46. Mader K, Gausepohl T, Pennig D. [Minimally invasive management of metacarpal I fractures with a mini-fixateur]. Handchir Mikrochir Plast Chir 2000; 32(2):107–11
47. McCulley SJ, Hasting C. External fixator for the hand: a quick, cheap and effective method. Journal of the Royal College of Surgeons of Edinburgh 1999;44(2): 99–102
48. Drenth DJ, Klasen HJ. External fixation for phalangeal and metacarpal fractures. The Journal of Bone and Joint Surgery 1998;80(2):227–30

Minimally Invasive Surgical Fixation of Distal Radius Fractures

14

Phani K. Dantuluri

The advent of improved surgical instrumentation and advances in healthcare have driven the rapidly evolving field of orthopedics. There has been a trend toward minimally invasive surgery in order to improve cosmesis, minimize soft tissue trauma, and allow superior fracture healing by minimally disturbing the biological environment around the fracture. Minimally invasive joint replacement surgery, arthroscopic surgery, and locking screw technology have been some of the newer developments in orthopedics that have significantly altered patient care and potentially the outcomes that can be achieved. In this regard, fractures of the distal radius have also been reexamined to see if minimally invasive surgery would be possible in treating this increasingly common fracture of the upper extremity and one of the leading reasons for visits to the emergency room.

Standard treatment for distal radius fractures not too long ago was cast immobilization. Closed reduction and percutaneous pinning and external fixation were some of the earlier methods used to treat fractures of the distal radius [1, 2]. However, there were limits to the types of fractures that could be treated closed, leading to increasing recognition of the importance of restoring articular congruity and fracture alignment [3, 4]. This needed to be done in an open fashion, and open reduction and internal fixation became much more common. Various types of plate and screw constructs were used to treat fractures of the distal radius. Plates were applied internally to the distal radius, as the idea of rigid fracture fixation with an internal implant was appealing to surgeon and patient alike [5].

This trend has accelerated rapidly over the last decade and, at this point, the most commonly used implant to treat fractures of the distal radius has become the volar plate [6]. Other pioneers in the field of upper extremity surgery have championed the cause of column-specific fixation with smaller implants addressing specific load-bearing areas of the distal radius in an attempt to provide more rigid fixation with smaller implants [7]. These methods have all been tremendously successful in treating fractures of the distal radius, however, problems still remain [8].

There is a thin soft tissue envelope surrounding the distal radius and the neurovascular structures are in very close proximity. Tendon and nerve complications are quite common with surgery of the distal radius despite advances in implant technology and lower profile implants [9, 10]. Locking screw technology has definitely improved fracture fixation and allowed for less complications as implants are lower profile, however, significant problems remain with tendon irritation and rupture as well as nerve problems, scar formation, stiffness, and the occasional need to remove implants.

P.K. Dantuluri (✉)
Department of Orthopaedics, Thomas Jefferson
University Hospital, Jefferson Medical College,
The Philadelphia Hand Center, Philadelphia, PA, USA
e-mail: pkdantuluri@handcenters.com

G.R. Scuderi and A.J. Tria (eds.), *Minimally Invasive Surgery in Orthopedics: Upper Extremity Handbook*,
DOI 10.1007/978-1-4614-0673-0_14, © Springer Science+Business Media, LLC 2012

The only type of implant that could potentially avoid these types of complications is an intramedullary one, as the implant could be seated completely underneath the cortical surface and not cause impingement on neighboring soft tissue and neurovascular structures. In addition, these implants can be inserted in the most minimally invasive fashion.

As modern medicine has rapidly surged forward, a greater understanding of the basic science of fracture healing has resulted. It has become clear that preservation of the blood supply to fracture fragments can greatly aid in fracture healing and lead to better clinical results. If one could successfully reduce a fracture and maintain its alignment with a minimal amount of soft tissue trauma while preserving the vascularity of fracture fragments, this would be optimal.

It has been known for quite some time that intramedullary implants have become the standard of care for diaphyseal fractures of the tibia and the femur in patients who need operative fixation [11]. These have been shown to have excellent results. The benefits of intramedullary fixation include less soft tissue trauma, preservation of the vascularity of fracture fragments, and an implant that acts as a load-sharing device rather than a load-bearing one. Some prior investigators have examined the concept of intramedullary fixation for fractures of the distal radius, but no specific completely intramedullary implant for the distal radius had been developed [12–19].

In an attempt to avoid many of the mentioned complications associated with the current surgical treatment of distal radius fractures, several investigators in conjunction with Wright Medical Technologies, Inc. have developed a novel intramedullary device (MICRONAIL) for fixation of distal radius fractures (Fig. 14.1). This implant utilizes fixed-angle locking screw technology in conjunction with an intramedullary construct in order to rigidly stabilize fractures of the distal radius while preserving fracture fragment vascularity and minimizing soft tissue trauma.

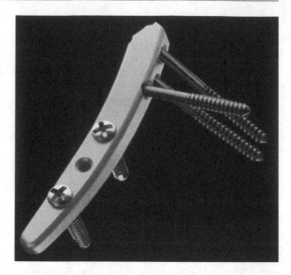

Fig. 14.1 MICRONAIL distributed by Wright Medical Technologies, Inc., demonstrating purple distal fixed-angle locking screws and gold proximal bicortical screws (From Dantuluri P. Distal Radius Fractures, An Issue of Atlas of the Hand Clinics, November 2006, with permission of Elsevier, Inc.)

Indications

Intramedullary nail fixation is best indicated for extraarticular distal radius fractures that are unstable and cannot be maintained with closed reduction (Fig. 14.2). Simple intraarticular fractures of the distal radius can also be treated with this device, but the fracture should have a minimum number of stable articular fragments and should not have extensive articular comminution. Fractures should also not have excessive metaphyseal-diaphyseal comminution with proximal extension, as the proximal fixation point for the device could be compromised, resulting in a loss of reduction. The device is an excellent choice for malunion surgery and is best indicated for extraarticular malunions of the distal radius. The device can provide an immediate rigid construct in malunion surgery and better disperse loading forces through the distal radius as it is a load-sharing device rather than a load-bearing one. This is of great benefit in malunion surgery as the resulting cortical defect that exists after surgical correction can take several months to reintegrate and, during this time, plate and screw constructs are subjected to tremendous loads that can lead to implant failure. It is necessary to carefully evaluate the initial injury and postreduction films to determine the appropriate patients amenable to intramedullary fixation.

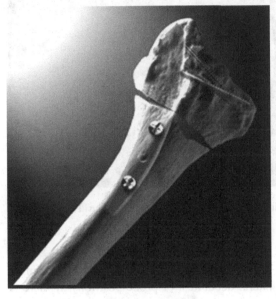

Fig. 14.2 Virtual image demonstrating ideal intramedullary nail position (From Dantuluri P. Distal Radius Fractures, An Issue of Atlas of the Hand Clinics, November 2006, with permission of Elsevier, Inc.)

Preoperative Planning

The preoperative radiographic evaluation follows a detailed history and physical examination and includes standard anteroposterior (AP), lateral, and oblique radiographs of the injured wrist (Fig. 14.3). Careful assessment of the ipsilateral upper extremity, particularly the elbow and forearm, are necessary to rule out more complex injury patterns, e.g., Essex-Lopresti injuries. Further radiographs of the forearm and elbow can be acquired if deemed necessary from the physical examination and history. A thorough neurovascular examination is of necessity and a careful assessment of the associated soft tissue injury is of paramount importance.

Contralateral radiographs of the opposite wrist are recommended in order to carefully evaluate each patient's individualized anatomy of the distal radius and are useful in preoperative templating

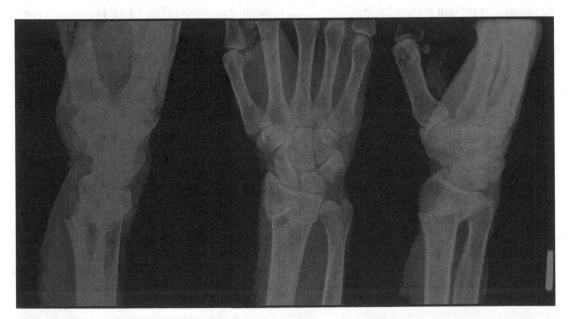

Fig. 14.3 Initial injury films demonstrating dorsal angulation, radial shortening, and loss of radial inclination (From Dantuluri P. Distal Radius Fractures, An Issue of Atlas of the Hand Clinics, November 2006, with permission of Elsevier, Inc.)

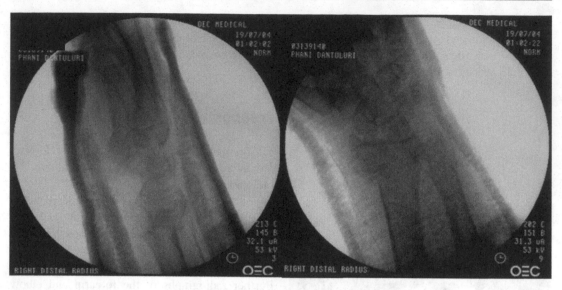

Fig. 14.4 Postreduction films demonstrate fracture instability and lack of alignment (From Dantuluri P. Distal Radius Fractures, An Issue of Atlas of the Hand Clinics, November 2006, with permission of Elsevier, Inc.)

for implant selection. Postreduction radiographs, if available, should also be evaluated to further assess fracture stability (Fig. 14.4). Prior history of injury or malunion of the injured distal radius needs to be addressed preoperatively as significant alteration in the normal parameters of the distal radius may prevent implant insertion.

Necessary Equipment

The minimally invasive surgical technique for intramedullary nail fixation of distal radius fractures described below requires the following specific equipment: (1) Wright Medical Intramedullary Implant System, (2) one 0.62 Kirshner wire and two 0.45 Kirshner wires, (3) K-wire driver, (4) drill, (5) small rongeur, and (6) intraoperative fluoroscopy.

Surgical Technique

Operative Setup

The versatility of the intramedullary system is that nail fixation can be performed if necessary in the multiply injured patient, in the supine, lateral decubitus, or prone positions. If there is no contraindication, surgery is most easily performed with the patient in the supine position. A standard arm board is attached to the side of the operating room table and is used to support the operative extremity (Fig. 14.5). However, a hand table can also alternatively be used, but the single arm board is the more versatile as it can be moved out of the way during the procedure when the fluoroscopic unit is in use. A mini-C arm fluoroscopy unit is preferred due to its decreased radiation exposure, but a standard fluoroscopy unit can be used as well.

Surgical Landmarks

Once the patient has been properly positioned and the arm prepped and draped in the usual sterile fashion, several key surgical landmarks should be identified. The radiocarpal and radioulnar joints should be palpated and identified. The tip and dorsal and volar contours of the radial styloid should also be identified. If excessive soft tissue swelling makes this difficult, fluoroscopy can be used to determine these critical landmarks and

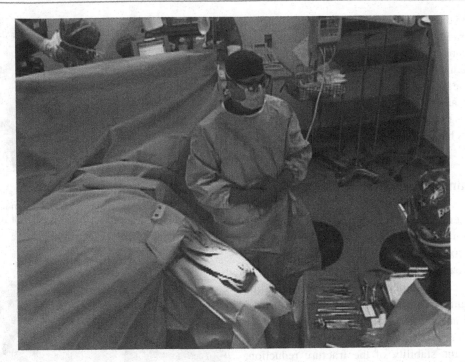

Fig. 14.5 Patient positioning with a single arm board for an injured extremity demonstrated (From Dantuluri P. Distal Radius Fractures, An Issue of Atlas of the Hand Clinics, November 2006, with permission of Elsevier, Inc.)

these areas can be marked on the skin to aid in the proper placement of surgical incisions.

Surgical Approach

Prior to the sterilely draped injured extremity being properly positioned on the arm board, the arm board should be adequately covered with a sterile drape, allowing the surgeon to grasp the arm board and move it without the risk of contamination. The fluoroscopic unit is then used to assess the fracture to confirm that it can easily be reduced or is able to be reduced with minimal percutaneous incisions. After it has been confirmed that the fracture can be reduced anatomically, the tip of the radial styloid is palpated and identified. A 2- to 3-cm longitudinal incision is then made centered over the tip of the radial styloid and midline between the dorsal and volar contours of the styloid (Fig. 14.6). Surgical dissection proceeds carefully at this point, and any branches of the radial sensory nerve that are in the field are identified and carefully retracted. No

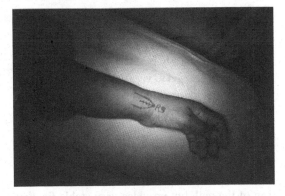

Fig. 14.6 Lateral view of injured extremity demonstrating contours of radial styloid (*RS*) and proposed surgical incision (From Dantuluri P. Distal Radius Fractures, An Issue of Atlas of the Hand Clinics, November 2006, with permission of Elsevier, Inc.)

skeletonization of these nerve branches should be done, and they should be retracted with their neighboring fat and vessels to avoid any radial sensory nerve problems postoperatively.

After the edges of the first and second dorsal extensor tendon compartments are identified, the periosteum between them is then incised in line with the skin incision, and the cortical surface of the radial styloid is exposed just enough for the entrance hole for the intramedullary nail. The periosteum should be preserved if possible so that it can be closed over the entrance hole later to prevent any adherence of the tendons or nerve branches to the nail underneath, which should be recessed below the cortical surface of the styloid.

Preliminary Reduction

It is of benefit to the surgeon to have an anatomic reduction of the fracture, which is held with K-wire fixation prior to nail insertion for a number of reasons. First, once the external jig is in place, it can be difficult to visualize the joint line and alignment of the fracture as both the jig and the nail are radio-opaque. Second, the nail may have a degree of intramedullary fill, which, while helping the stability of the fracture reduction, can prevent any fine tuning of the reduction once the implant is in place, particularly in terms of dorsal or volar translation or restoration of volar tilt. Thus, it is recommended that the fracture be anatomically reduced and held prior to nail insertion.

This can generally be easily done and fluoroscopy should be used to verify the anatomic reduction. Once the fracture is reduced, the distal fragment is then preliminarily pinned with a 0.62 K-wire inserted through the radial styloid with fixation in the shaft proximally. This K-wire should inserted, if possible, in the volar portion of the styloid so that it will not interfere with insertion of the nail, but provides very stable fixation of the distal fragment and also helps to protect and retract the tendons of the first dorsal extensor compartment and sensory branches of the radial sensory nerve (Fig. 14.7). This can be a difficult K-wire to insert, but is well worth the effort as it makes the rest of the procedure much easier.

A second percutaneous 0.45 K-wire is then inserted dorsally, typically between the fourth and fifth dorsal extensor compartments. A small 1-mm stab incision can be made here to ensure that the correct interval has been entered and that the K-wire does not entangle tendons or sensory

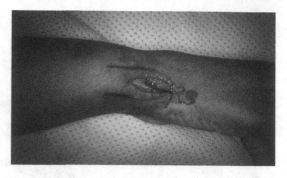

Fig. 14.7 Demonstration of surgical exposure and placement of 0.62 K-wire volarly in the styloid (From Dantuluri P. Distal Radius Fractures, An Issue of Atlas of the Hand Clinics, November 2006, with permission of Elsevier, Inc.)

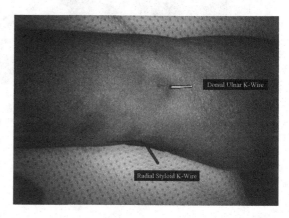

Fig. 14.8 Preliminary reduction maintained with dorsal ulnar and radial styloid K-wires providing rigid 90/90 fixation (From Dantuluri P. Distal Radius Fractures, An Issue of Atlas of the Hand Clinics, November 2006, with permission of Elsevier, Inc.)

nerve branches. Typically, a guide can be slid down over the K-wire once it is in the proper 4–5 interval prior to insertion to prevent any soft tissues from wrapping around the wire. This K-wire should capture the dorsal ulnar corner of the distal fragment and, in conjunction with the 0.62 K-wire through the radial styloid, provide rigid 90/90 fixation of the distal fragment (Fig. 14.8).

It is recommended to achieve this anatomic rigid 90/90 fixation prior to nail insertion, as while insertion of the nail should be a gentle process, it can disrupt the preliminary reduction if inadequate K-wire fixation is achieved. The rigid 90/90 fixation provided by the two K-wires best

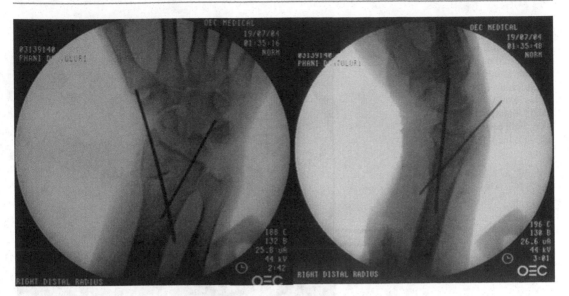

Fig. 14.9 Fluoroscopic images demonstrating typical K-wire positions to maintain preliminary reduction. Note volar position of 0.62 K-wire in the lateral view and note the dorsal ulnar position of the 0.45 K-wire in the posteroanterior (PA) (From Dantuluri P. Distal Radius Fractures, An Issue of Atlas of the Hand Clinics, November 2006, with permission of Elsevier, Inc.)

resists any displacement forces created through the nail insertion process (Fig. 14.9).

If the reduction of the fracture cannot be achieved by closed means, one can utilize the anticipated small dorsal incision for the proximal locking screws as a window to help with the reduction without making any additional incisions. The nail can be placed on the dorsal surface of the skin in its expected intramedullary position with the wrist in a posteroanterior position on the fluoroscopic unit. Fluoroscopy will reveal the anticipated incision site for the proximal locking screws. A Freer elevator can then be inserted through this incision to help reduce difficult fractures, particularly in the region of the sigmoid notch as well as simple articular fractures. Once reduction has been achieved, the K-wires should be inserted as previously described.

Nail Insertion

At this point, the tip of the radial styloid is identified and a cortical window is made in the styloid approximately 5 mm proximal to the tip of the styloid. This cortical window must be made proximal enough in the styloid to prevent violation of the articular surface of the scaphoid facet with successive broaching, but not be too proximal to prevent adequate subchondral support with the distal locking screws. An awl or the 6.1 cannulated drill bit can be used to make this entrance hole in the styloid (Fig. 14.10). Fluoroscopy should be used at this critical step to ensure the proper entrance hole for insertion of the intramedullary implant.

After the cortical window has been made, a small rongeur can be used to expand the window typically in the proximal direction longitudinally in line with the radius for about 5 mm in order to allow atraumatic broach insertion. A small canal finder is then inserted gently into the intramedullary canal (Fig. 14.11). It is critical that the canal finder should stay along the radial cortex during insertion in order to prevent penetration of the ulnar cortex of the radial shaft. Using fluoroscopy to ensure proper entry, a small broach is then inserted across the fracture site and advanced proximally across the metaphyseal-diaphyseal junction (Fig. 14.12). Increasingly larger broaches are then inserted sequentially until the broach is large enough within the canal to resist spinning

Fig. 14.10 Guide wire placed in tip of styloid for cannulated drill insertion to create entrance hole for implant (From Dantuluri P. Distal Radius Fractures, An Issue of Atlas of the Hand Clinics, November 2006, with permission of Elsevier, Inc.)

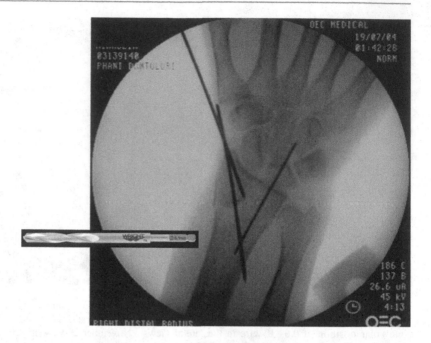

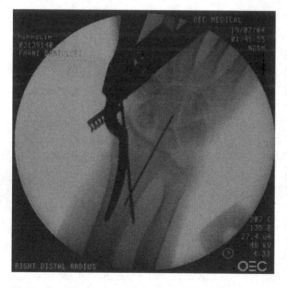

Fig. 14.11 Canal finder insertion. Note that the canal finder hugs the radial cortex to prevent ulnar cortical perforation (From Dantuluri P. Distal Radius Fractures, An Issue of Atlas of the Hand Clinics, November 2006, with permission of Elsevier, Inc.)

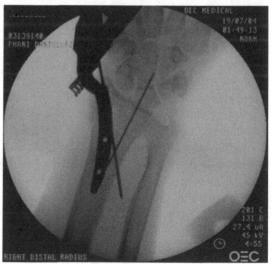

Fig. 14.12 Broach insertion demonstrating an expected position of the intramedullary nail (From Dantuluri P. Distal Radius Fractures, An Issue of Atlas of the Hand Clinics, November 2006, with permission of Elsevier, Inc.)

when rotational torque is applied as well provide reasonable intramedullary fill. Preoperative templating using the contralateral wrist radiographs should also provide the surgeon with valuable information as to which size implant is the likely size that will be used.

After the last broach has been removed, the implant is then mounted on the external jig and then gently inserted following the path of the prior broach (Fig. 14.13). The nail should be carefully inserted toward the sigmoid notch far enough medially into the radius so that no part of

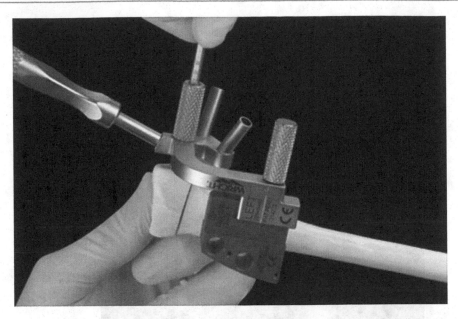

Fig. 14.13 Close up view of external jig demonstrating screw alignment guides for proximal and distal screw insertion in sawbones model (From Dantuluri P. Distal Radius Fractures, An Issue of Atlas of the Hand Clinics, November 2006, with permission of Elsevier, Inc.)

the nail is protruding above the radial cortex (Fig. 14.14). This will prevent any contact between the nail and the undersurface of the tendons of either the first or second compartment. In addition, the nail is inserted gently proximally enough so that the distal-most locking screw will be just underneath the subchondral bone supporting the radiocarpal articular surface. A K-wire or a drill bit can be inserted through the distal-most drill guide and then checked under fluoroscopy to ensure that the distal-most locking screw will be in the desired subchondral position (Fig. 14.15).

At this point, the distal locking screw holes are drilled and measured and three distal locking screws are inserted into the nail with the distal-most screw inserted first (Fig. 14.16). Fluoroscopy should also be used when measuring the length of the screws to ensure that they do not penetrate the sigmoid notch and enter the distal radioulnar joint (Fig. 14.17). It is important to remember that the sigmoid notch has a concavity for the distal ulna so that a screw may appear to be safely out of the distal radial ulnar joint on the fluoroscopic view, but may still actually be penetrating this joint. Therefore, it is best to have these screws err on the side of being 2 mm short and be sure to check for crepitus. Once all of the distal locking screws

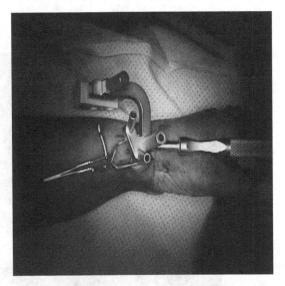

Fig. 14.14 External jig in place with intramedullary nail insertion (From Dantuluri P. Distal Radius Fractures, An Issue of Atlas of the Hand Clinics, November 2006, with permission of Elsevier, Inc.)

have firmly locked into the nail, the fracture reduction should be carefully assessed (Fig. 14.18). If there has been a slight loss of reduction of the fracture due to nail insertion, an attempt can now be made to gently reduce the fracture anatomically prior to proximal screw insertion.

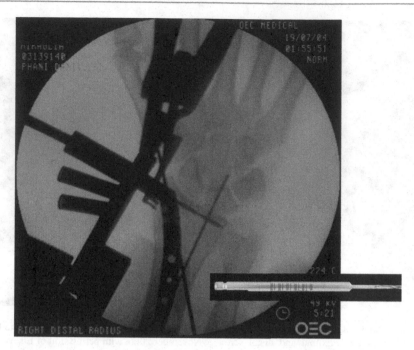

Fig. 14.15 Drilling of distal locking screws with care to avoid penetration of radiocarpal and radioulnar joints (From Dantuluri P. Distal Radius Fractures, An Issue of Atlas of the Hand Clinics, November 2006, with permission of Elsevier, Inc.)

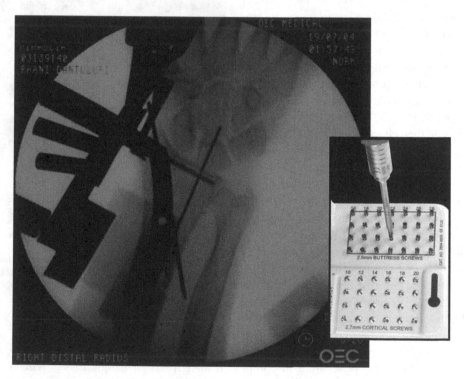

Fig. 14.16 Distal locking screw insertion (From Dantuluri P. Distal Radius Fractures, An Issue of Atlas of the Hand Clinics, November 2006, with permission of Elsevier, Inc.)

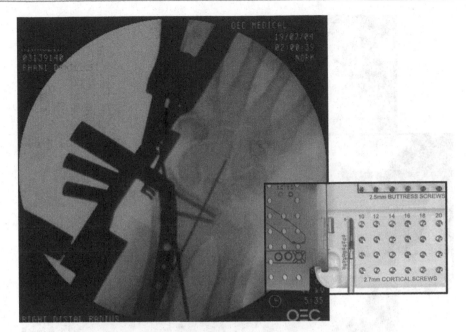

Fig. 14.17 Insertion of remaining distal locking screws keeping them short of the sigmoid notch to avoid penetration (From Dantuluri P. Distal Radius Fractures, An Issue of Atlas of the Hand Clinics, November 2006, with permission of Elsevier, Inc.)

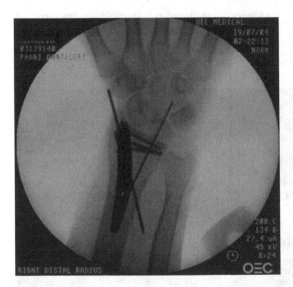

Fig. 14.18 Fluoroscopic image after completed distal locking screw insertion demonstrating ideal distal locking screw positions (From Dantuluri P. Distal Radius Fractures, An Issue of Atlas of the Hand Clinics, November 2006, with permission of Elsevier, Inc.)

At this stage, a 0.45 K-wire is then inserted through the dorsal cortex and the nail to rigidly hold the implant in place and prevent subtle displacement of the implant within the canal or loss of reduction. The proximal screws can then be inserted through two small 1-cm incisions or one single 2-cm dorsal incision. The appropriate drill guide and sleeves are used to drill and insert the proximal screws (Fig. 14.19). These screws achieve bicortical purchase and lock the implant in place. It is important to prevent any soft tissue such as extensor tendons from being trapped under the screw heads. Also, it is *critical* not to compromise purchase of the proximal locking screws by overtightening as there are only two proximal locking screws and they are crucial in maintaining implant position and proximal fixation, especially if there is not good intramedullary fill of the implant. A good technique to avoid stripping these screws is retracting the drill guides for the last few turns so that this can done under direct visualization so that it is clear when the screw heads are down tight on the dorsal cortex of the radius.

Final fluoroscopic images are used to verify that the reduction of the fracture has been accomplished and that the implant and all screws are in appropriate positions (Fig. 14.20). The periosteum is then closed over the cortical window in the radial styloid if possible to prevent any contact of

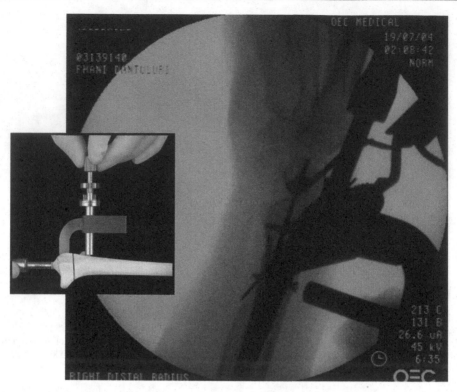

Fig. 14.19 Proximal locking insertion demonstrating how the drill guide can be withdrawn for the final few turns to allow direct visualization and avoid stripping of the screws (From Dantuluri P. Distal Radius Fractures, An Issue of Atlas of the Hand Clinics, November 2006, with permission of Elsevier, Inc.)

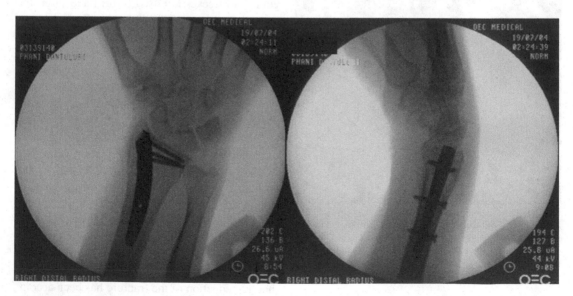

Fig. 14.20 Completed intramedullary fixation of distal radius fracture demonstrating anatomic reduction and ideal implant placement (From Dantuluri P. Distal Radius Fractures, An Issue of Atlas of the Hand Clinics, November 2006, with permission of Elsevier, Inc.)

the nail with the surrounding soft tissues. The deeper subcutaneous tissues are closed with a minimum of 2.0 Vicryl suture and the skin is closed with 3.0 Monocryl subcuticular suture (Fig. 14.21). Benzoin and Steri-strips are then applied and patient's arm is placed into a temporary short arm splint for comfort.

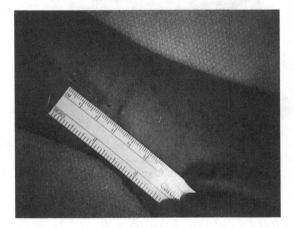

Fig. 14.21 Postoperative closure demonstrating 2-cm incision for nail insertion (From Dantuluri P. Distal Radius Fractures, An Issue of Atlas of the Hand Clinics, November 2006, with permission of Elsevier, Inc.)

Postoperative Care

Patients are instructed to begin immediate postoperative finger, elbow, and shoulder range of motion to avoid stiffness and reduce swelling. Patients are typically seen for their first postoperative visit at a week to 10 days. At that visit, they are given a removable orthoplast short arm splint only for comfort. At this point, unrestricted active range of motion is allowed for the wrist as well and patients are also instituted in occupational therapy to monitor and aid in their rehabilitation. Patients are followed with serial radiographs to evaluate bony union, which typically occurs at approximately 6 weeks postoperatively (Fig. 14.22). New developments in the instrumentation system include the development of longer intramedullary nails (Fig. 14.23) to provide better proximal fixation. Having three proximal screws allows superior fixation of the implant and prevents proximal migration of the nail (Figs. 14.24 and 14.25). The most significant new development is the introduction of a radiolucent guide, which allows better visualization of the fracture lines, allowing superior fracture reductions (Fig. 14.26). In this example case, one

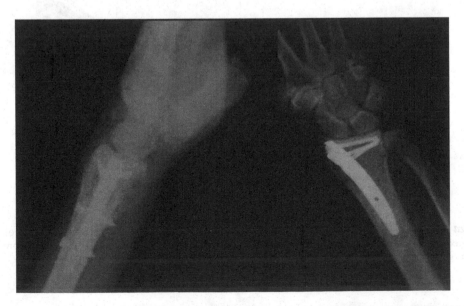

Fig. 14.22 Early postoperative radiographs demonstrating maintenance of reduction (From Dantuluri P. Distal Radius Fractures, An Issue of Atlas of the Hand Clinics, November 2006, with permission of Elsevier, Inc.)

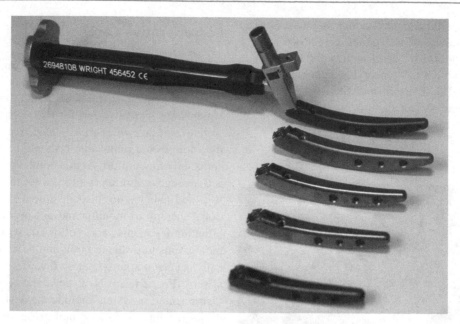

Fig. 14.23 New developments in intramedullary nail fixation include longer intramedullary nails allowing better proximal fixation (From Dantuluri P. Distal Radius Fractures, An Issue of Atlas of the Hand Clinics, November 2006, with permission of Elsevier, Inc.)

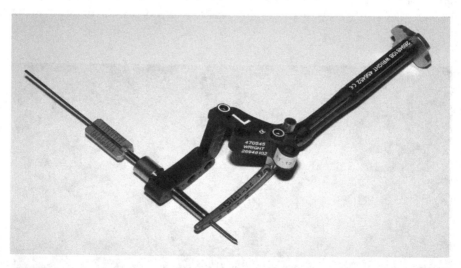

Fig. 14.24 Improved proximal fixation is allowed by having three proximal screws that engage the distal radius and also go through the intramedullary nail (From Dantuluri P. Distal Radius Fractures, An Issue of Atlas of the Hand Clinics, November 2006, with permission of Elsevier, Inc.)

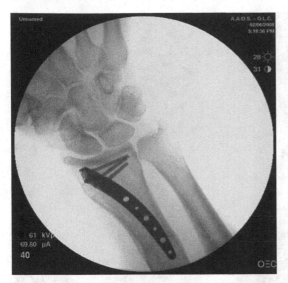

Fig. 14.25 Example of newer intramedullary design with implant in place demonstrating the three proximal screw fixation points (From Dantuluri P. Distal Radius Fractures, An Issue of Atlas of the Hand Clinics, November 2006, with permission of Elsevier, Inc.)

can see the superior visualization afforded by the radiolucent guide of the distal radius, particularly on the lateral view, allowing anatomic reductions of both the radiocarpal and distal radioulnar joints (Fig. 14.27).

Follow-Up Results and Complications

It has been shown, at least in short-term follow-up, that distal radius fractures can be successfully treated with intramedullary fixation. Tan et al. presented a prospective study of 23 consecutive fractures treated with intramedullary fixation using the MICRONAIL [20]. This study showed that outcomes were excellent at 6-month follow-up in terms of maintenance of alignment of the distal radius, range of motion, and improvement of grip strength. Outcome measurements using standardized outcome tools (DASH) also demonstrated excellent results. There were relatively

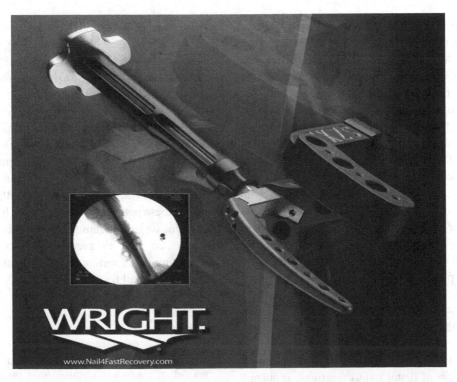

Fig. 14.26 Development of a new radiolucent guide allows superior visualization of the fracture and allows more precise placement of the distal and proximal screws (From Dantuluri P. Distal Radius Fractures, An Issue of Atlas of the Hand Clinics, November 2006, with permission of Elsevier, Inc.)

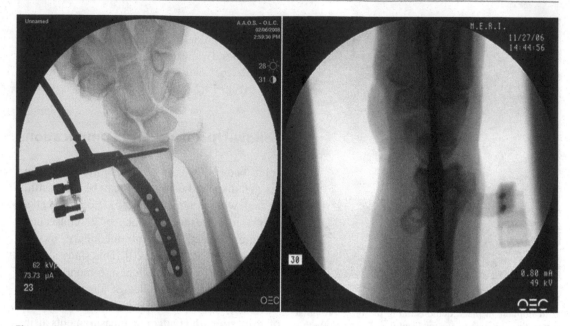

Fig. 14.27 Example of the radiolucent guide in place demonstrating the views afforded of the distal radius. Much more of the bony landmarks of the distal radius can be visualized with the radiolucent guide, which will allow for superior fracture reductions and exact screw placement (From Dantuluri P. Distal Radius Fractures, An Issue of Atlas of the Hand Clinics, November 2006, with permission of Elsevier, Inc.)

few complications and these consisted of three transient radial sensory nerve injuries, and three patients who had loss of fracture reduction, but these patients all had more complex intraarticular fracture types. As with any surgical implant, improperly measured screws can lead to soft tissue complications or loss of reduction. Screws not placed just underneath the articular surface of the distal radius can result in possible fracture subsidence and loss of alignment. Penetration of either the radiocarpal or radioulnar joints with screws can lead to irreversible articular damage. It is clear in early follow-up that intramedullary fixation of distal radius fractures is not only possible, but can lead to excellent results in properly selected patients [21].

Significant scarring of tendons and neurovascular structures can occur with extensive surgical dissection, leading to limitation of function. The thin soft tissue envelope surrounding the distal radius and the close proximity of tendons, nerves, and vascular structures to the distal radius may contribute to the development of some of these complications. Minimally invasive surgical fixation of the distal radius has been developed using an intramedullary nail as a new treatment option for fractures of the distal radius in an attempt to minimize these potential complications. It is clear that careful surgical technique and proper patient selection can lead to successful outcomes in patients with distal radius fractures treated with intramedullary nail fixation [21].

Conclusions

Despite the success of open reduction and internal fixation of distal radius fractures, problems persist, including loss of reduction, hardware failure, tendon and nerve injuries, and infection.

References

1. Simic P, Weiland A. Fractures of the distal aspect of the radius; changes in treatment over the past two decades. *J Bone Joint Surg (Am)* 2003;85:552–564
2. McQuuen MM. Redisplaced unstable fractures of the distal radius. A randomized prospective study of

bridging versus non-bridging external fixation. *J Bone Joint Surg* 1998;80B:665–669

3. Knirk JL, Jupiter JB. Intraarticular fractures of the distal end of the radius in young adults. *J Bone Joint Surg* 1986;68:647–659

4. Lafontaine M, Hardy D, Delince P. Stability assessment in distal radius fractures. *Injury* 1989;20:208–210

5. Ruch DS, Papadonikolakis A. Volar versus dorsal plating in the management of intraarticular distal radius fractures. *J Hand Surg (Am)* 2006;31(1):9–16

6. Orbay JL, Fernandez DL. Volar fixed-angle plate fixation for unstable distal radius fractures in the elderly patient. *J Hand Surg* 2004;29:96–102

7. Ring D, Prommersberger K, Jupiter JB. Combined dorsal and volar plate fixation of complex fractures of the distal part of the radius. *J Bone Joint Surg Am* 2004;86:1646–1652

8. Jakob M, Rikli DA, Regazzoni P. Fracture of the distal radius treated by internal fixation and early function. A prospective study of 73 consecutive patients. *J Bone Joint Surg* 2000;82:340–344

9. Rozental TD, Beredjiklian PK, Bozentka DJ. Functional outcome and complications following two types of dorsal plating for unstable fractures of the distal part of the radius. *J Bone Joint Surg Am* 2003; 85:1956–1960

10. Rozental TD, Blazar PE. Functional outcome and complications after volar plating for dorsally displaced, unstable fractures of the distal radius. *J Hand Surg (Am)* 2006;31(3):359–365

11. Tarr RR, Wiss DA. The mechanics and biology of intramedullary fracture fixation. *Clin Orthop Relat Res* 1986;212:10–17

12. Pritchett JW. External fixation or closed medullary pinning for unstable Colles' fractures? *J Bone Joint Surg* 1995;77:267–269

13. Saeki Y, Hashizume H, Nagoshi M, Tanaka H, Inoue H. Mechanical strength of intramedullary pinning and transfragmental Kirschner wire fixation for Colles' fractures. *J Hand Surg (Br)* 2001;26:550–555

14. Sato O, Aoki M, Kawaguchi S, Ishii S, Kondo M. Antegrade intramedullary K-wire fixation for distal radius fractures. *J Hand Surg* 2002;27:707–713

15. Street DM. Intramedullary forearm nailing. *Clin Orthop Relat Res* 1986;212:219–230

16. Van der Reis WL, Otsuka NY, Moroz P, et al. Intramedullary nailing versus plate fixation for unstable forearm fractures in children. *J Pediatr Orthop* 1998;18:9–13

17. Gao H, Luo CF, Zhang CO, Shi HP, Fan CY, Zen BF. Internal fixation of diaphyseal fractures of the forearm by interlocking intramedullary nail: short term result in eighteen patients. *J Orthop Trauma* 2005;19(6): 384–391

18. Sasaki S. Modified Desmanet's intramedullary pinning for fractures of the distal radius. *J Orthop Sci* 2002;7(2):172–181

19. Bennett GL, Leeson MC, Smith BS. Intramedullary fixation of unstable distal radius fractures: a method of fixation allowing early motion. *Orthop Rev* 1989;18(2):210–216

20. Tan V, Capo JT, Warburton M. Distal radius fracture fixation with an intramedullary nail. *Tech Hand Up Extrem Surg* 2005;9(4):195–201

21. Brooks KR, Capo JT, Warburton M, Tan V. Internal fixation of distal radius fractures with novel intramedullary implants. *Clin Orthop Relat Res* 2006 Apr;(445): 42–50

Minimally Invasive Fixation for Wrist Fractures

15

Louis W. Catalano III, Milan M. Patel, and Steven Z. Glickel

There are multiple techniques for treating distal radius fractures. Closed reduction and percutaneous pinning remains a valid and well-accepted method of surgical treatment for displaced and unstable fractures. Pinning has been described for both intraarticular and extraarticular fractures and it represents a relatively simple, minimally invasive, and cost-effective method of treatment. This technique may become more appealing as complications from volar plating are being reported in the literature.

Indications and Contraindications

The goal of surgical treatment of distal radius fractures is to obtain and maintain anatomic reduction in order to maximize the patient's functional outcome. Percutaneous pinning can be used for both extraarticular (AO/ASIF type A2 and A3) and intraarticular fractures, including three- and four-part fractures (AO/ASIF type C1 and C2). Pinning is most effective for fractures that can be closed reduced by traction, manipulation, and ligamentotaxis. Contraindications for percutaneous pinning alone (without augmentation, using external fixation or open reduction

L.W. Catalano III (✉)
Department of Orthopaedic Surgery, Columbia College of Physicians and Surgeons, New York, NY, USA

C.V. Starr Hand Surgery Center, St. Luke's-Roosevelt Hospital Center, New York, NY, USA
e-mail: catalano@msn.com

and internal fixation) include severe metaphyseal or intraarticular comminution (AO/ASIF type C3), poor bone stock, and shear fractures (AO/ASIF type B). Fixation of these fractures with percutaneous pinning can lead to loss of reduction and subsequent malunions.

Techniques for Radial Pinning

Several techniques of percutaneous pinning of distal radius fractures have been described in the literature. Techniques of radial pinning have included one or multiple pins placed obliquely through the radial styloid (Fig. 15.1a), crossed pinning from the radial styloid and dorsoulnar cortex (Fig. 15.1b), intrafocal pinning within the distal radius fracture site (Fig. 15.1c), and oblique and horizontal pins placed through the radial styloid (Fig. 15.2). In 1907, Lambotte [1] described using a single radial styloid pin as a method of stabilization, and in 1959, Willenegger and Guggenbuhl [2] further reported on their experience with this method in 25 patients. In 1975, Stein and Katz [3], and in 1984, Clancey [4] described crossed pinning of the radius, using one or more pins through the radial styloid and another pin through the dorsal and ulnar corner of the distal radius. This technique stabilized the dorsoulnar radial fragment and provided orthogonal pin configuration, inherently more stable than pins in one plane. Fernandez and Geissler [5] described another method for stabilizing the dorsoulnar fragment. In addition to two oblique

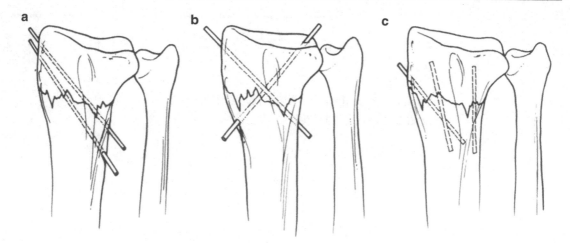

Fig. 15.1 (a) Multiple pins placed obliquely through the radial styloid. (b) Crossing pins from the radial styloid and dorsoulnar corner. (c) Intrafocal pinning into the distal radius fracture (From Fernandez DL, Jupiter JB. Fractures of the Distal Radius. A Practical Approach to Management, 2nd ed., New York: Springer, 2002, p. 153, with kind permission of Springer Science and Business Media)

radial styloid pins, they placed transverse pins in the subchondral bone from the radial styloid to the ulnar fragment, avoiding entering the distal radioulnar joint (DRUJ). The transverse pin supported the intraarticular fracture fragments, preventing displacement. In 1976, Kapandji [6] reported a technique of intrafocal pinning using two pins in the fracture site for reduction and buttress fixation of the fracture and modified this in 1987, using three-pin intrafocal pinning [7].

Practically, these techniques of closed reduction and percutaneous pinning are used alone or in combination depending on the particular fracture pattern. The number of pins, size of the pins, and configuration within the distal radius are adapted to the fracture pattern. In a biomechanical study, Naidu et al. [8] demonstrated that crossed pinning with at least 0.062-in.-diameter K-wires was more rigid than two parallel radial styloid pins alone. Rogge et al. [9] corroborated this finding in their study using mathematical and computer-generated finite element modeling. Our approach and technique is described below.

A pneumatic tourniquet is placed on the arm and the hand and arm are prepped and draped with a stockinette and a prefabricated extremity drape. The procedure is performed using a radiolucent hand table to which an outrigger for longitudinal traction can be incorporated. We currently use the Carter hand surgery table (Innovation Sport, Foothill Ranch, CA) for the traction set-up. Finger traps on the index and long fingers are attached to a wire, which runs over the pulley of the traction outrigger. Depending on the size of the patient, five or ten pounds of weight are applied for longitudinal traction with the limb horizontal on the hand table (Fig. 15.3). The head and arm of the image intensifier are sterilely draped. The image intensifier is brought into the operative field and posteroanterior (PA) and lateral images of the distal radius are obtained. The fracture is manipulated with volarly directed pressure on the dorsum of the distal fracture fragment in an effort to restore length and volar tilt. Volar tilt can also be regained by translating the carpus volarly. In instances where the distal fracture fragment is radially translated, ulnarly directed pressure on the radial styloid and/or ulnar translation of the wrist by ulnar deviation and manual translation of the hand can facilitate reduction. The reduction is monitored fluoroscopically. If it is thought that reduction is achievable, the surgeon proceeds with the planned percutaneous pin fixation. If the fracture is not reducible closed, open reduction and internal fixation may be required.

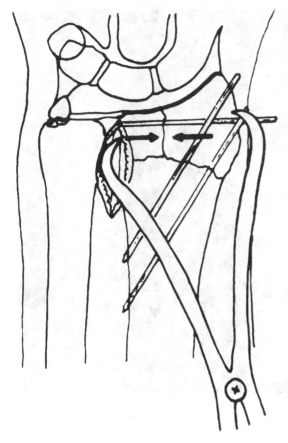

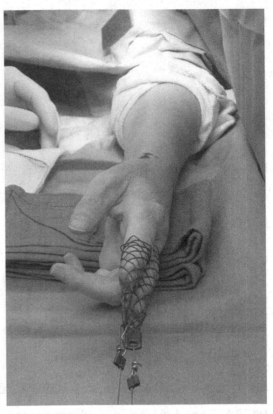

Fig. 15.3 Fingertraps are placed on the index and middle fingers. Ten pounds of traction is placed through the fingertraps to aid with the reduction and to keep the fracture out to length

Fig. 15.2 Multiple pins placed obliquely through the radial styloid are combined with transverse pins to capture the dorsoulnar radial fragment. Subchondral pins can also help buttress the depressed lunate facet. The dorsoulnar radial fragment can be reduced through a small incision utilizing a bone tenaculum (From Fernandez DL, Jupiter JB. Fractures of the Distal Radius. A Practical Approach to Management, 2nd ed., New York: Springer, 2002, p. 153, with kind permission of Springer Science and Business Media)

Fractures treated 2–3 weeks after injury may be difficult to reduce simply with manipulation and manual pressure (Fig. 15.4). In that case, an intrafocal pin may be used to assist in the reduction. If the fracture is shortened and the distal articular surface dorsally tilted, an intrafocal pin is placed into the fracture dorsally at an angle from proximal to distal. The position of the pin is confirmed fluoroscopically and the pin is used to manually advance the distal fracture fragment distally and volarly by levering the pin distally, changing the obliquity of the pin from distal to

proximal. Usually, this can be done percutaneously. The exception is a fracture close to 3-weeks old that is healed enough that a 0.062-in. K-wire is not sufficiently rigid to accomplish the goal of mobilization of the distal fracture fragment. In that case, a small Freer elevator can be used percutaneously in the same manner (Fig. 15.5a, b). An intrafocal wire can than be placed from dorsal to volar in order to maintain the reduction that was created by breaking up the healing callus.

A similar intrafocal technique can be used to restore loss of radial inclination. This should be done under direct vision to avoid injury to the superficial radial nerve and the tendons of the first compartment. A 0.062-in. K-wire is placed into the fracture at an angle from proximal to distal. The pin is levered distally, forcing the fracture fragment distally as well as translating it ulnarly.

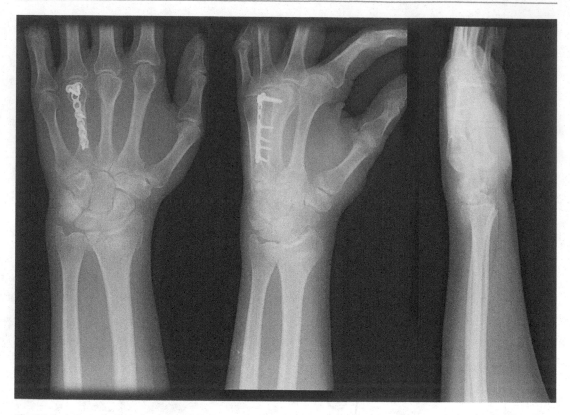

Fig. 15.4 A 3-week-old displaced distal radius fracture in a 50-year old man that is amenable to minimally invasive fixation

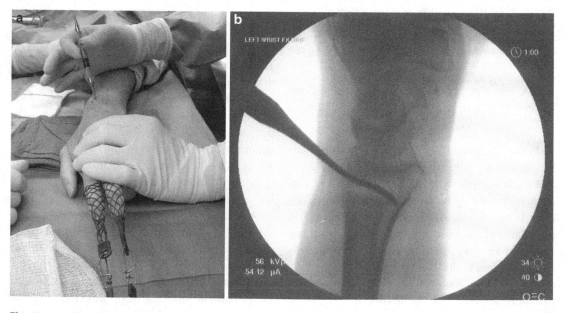

Fig. 15.5 (a, b) A small elevator is placed through a stab incision into the fracture site to aid with restoration of the normal volar tilt of the distal radius

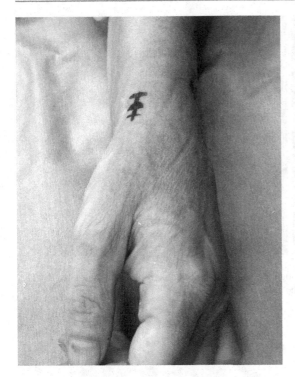

Fig. 15.6 The incision to identify the superficial radial nerve and first dorsal compartment is marked out at the radial styloid

Once the reduction is felt to be satisfactory, percutaneous pin fixation is achieved using the technique described previously. The surgeon may opt to leave the intrafocal pin in place and drive it proximally into the ulnar cortex of the radius, proximal to the fracture site. This intrafocal K-wire helps prevent loss of radial inclination, which can produce irritating cosmetic concerns for the patient.

Our preference is to place 2–3 pins from the radial styloid. The pins are 0.062-in. in diameter. We place the pins under direct vision in order to avoid injury to the superficial radial nerve or the tendons of the first dorsal compartment. A 1.5-cm-long longitudinal incision is made extending from the tip of the radial styloid distally (Fig. 15.6). The superficial radial nerve is identified and retracted. The pins are usually placed just dorsal to the first extensor compartment but may be placed volar to the compartment depending upon the pattern of the fracture and the location of the nerve. There is frequently some loss of

reduction of the fracture once manual pressure on the distal fracture fragment is released in order to begin pin placement. Therefore, the first pin is placed in the distal fracture fragment, not crossing the fracture line. The pin is always placed through a soft tissue protector in order to avoid wrapping up adjacent soft tissues structures. The first pin is started at the tip of the radial styloid and directed at a fairly shallow angle obliquely, with the goal of crossing the fracture line and engaging the ulnar cortex of the radius proximal to the fracture. Once the pin is driven into the distal fracture fragment with a K-wire driver, the fracture is re-reduced and the reduction confirmed with PA and lateral radiographs. When the fracture is anatomically reduced, the K-wire is driven across the fracture and the distal radial metaphysis engaging the ulnar cortex proximal to the fracture line. Postfixation fluoroscopic images are obtained (Fig. 15.7a, b). Usually, a second 0.062-in. K-wire is placed at a slightly more proximal starting point and at a slightly different angle than the initial pin, directing it more dorsally or volarly within the medullary canal and aiming more proximally (Fig. 15.8a, b). Reduction and fixation are confirmed with the image intensifier.

For two-part fractures, another set of pins is placed perpendicular to the radial styloid pins. Generally, we place those pins beginning from the dorsal rim of the distal radius just distal to Lister's tubercle. The pins should be started just distal to the tubercle or slightly radial to it. Beginning the pin ulnar to that point runs the risk of tethering or otherwise injuring the extensor pollicis longus (EPL) tendon. The wrist is placed in position to obtain a lateral image and the starting point of the pin at the dorsal rim of the radius is confirmed (Fig. 15.9). The authors find it easier to manually insert the K-wire and feel the dense, solid dorsal rim of the distal radius. It is important to start the pin in the solid bone of the dorsal rim of the radius as opposed to the more proximal metaphyseal region where the cortex is thinner and may be comminuted from the fracture. The pin is driven obliquely from dorsal to volar across the fracture line, engaging the volar cortex of the radius proximal to the fracture. In some patients,

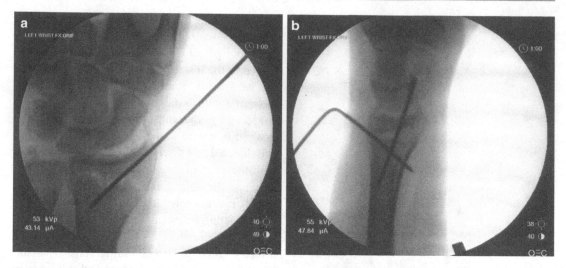

Fig. 15.7 (a) A 0.062-in. K-wire is placed obliquely through the radial styloid and across the fracture site. (b) The second K-wire is driven as an intrafocal wire to maintain the volar tilt

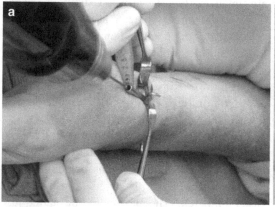
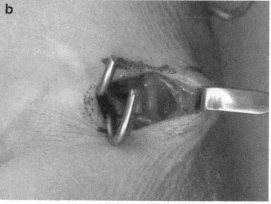

Fig. 15.8 (a) A second oblique wire is placed through the radial styloid at a slightly different angle and a soft tissue protector is used to avoid wrapping up the adjacent structures. (b) The radial styloid incision with the obliquely directed K-wires and an adjacent superficial vein and the superficial radial nerve

a second pin may be placed in a similar manner beginning just proximal to the first pin and directed at a slightly different angle to enhance the fixation.

Some modifications of this basic pinning technique are used in specific fractures to assist with the reduction or provide fixation for the ulnar fracture fragment in three-part fractures. If the fracture has three parts and there is any proximal subsidence of the lunate fossa creating a step off, this may be addressed percutaneously as well.

If there is proximal displacement of the lunate fossa fragment, it can be advanced distally using an intrafocal pin placed percutaneously into the dorsum of the fracture as described previously. The pin is angled from proximal to distal and the fracture fragment advanced distally as the pin is pushed in an arc from proximal to distal. Fixation of the lunate fossa fragment can be achieved in one of two ways. Proximal subsidence of the fracture can be prevented by placing two transverse pins from the radial styloid across the distal radial

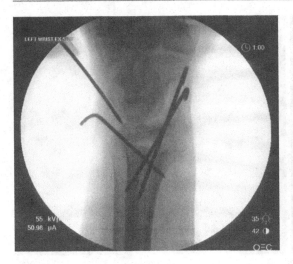

Fig. 15.9 Another perpendicular 0.062-in. K-wire is placed from just distal to Lister's tubercle starting on the solid bone of the dorsal rim

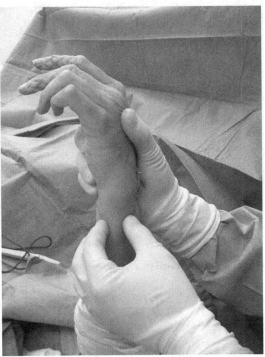

Fig. 15.10 The DRUJ is tested for instability after the fixation of the radius is finalized

metaphysis just proximal to the subchondral bone (see Fig. 15.2). One pin is placed volarly and the other pin is placed dorsally across the distal radius. The tips of the pins are driven to engage the ulnar cortex of the radius in the area of the sigmoid notch but the pins should not extend beyond the cortex into the DRUJ. An alternative is to fix the lunate fossa fragment with a pin placed percutaneously from the dorsoulnar corner of the distal radius, driving it obliquely in a dorsovolar direction to engage the volar cortex proximal to the fracture line. In general, that pin is started in the interval between the fourth and fifth extensor compartments and the starting point of the pin is confirmed fluoroscopically prior to advancing the pin.

Once the distal radius fracture is stabilized, the DRUJ is examined to assess stability (Fig. 15.10). If the joint is unstable, and there is no ulnar styloid fracture, the DRUJ is stabilized by pinning the ulna to the radius with two 0.062-in. Kirscher wires placed transversely proximal to the joint. If the ulnar styloid is fractured at its base, consideration is given to fixing the fracture using a tension band construct.

The reduction and fixation is assessed with final fluoroscopic images in at least two planes (Fig. 15.11a, b). The pins are left superficial to

the skin and are bent using pliers to prevent migration. The radial styloid pins may be left through the incision. If the K-wires tent the skin, the skin either needs to be released with a secondary incision or the pin can be cut and, before bending it, placed through the skin adjacent to the incision obviating the need for relaxing incisions. The radial styloid incision is closed with interrupted absorbable sutures thereby precluding suture removal.

Postoperative Care and Rehabilitation

The fracture is usually immobilized for the first 2 weeks postoperatively in a sugar tong splint. It is our impression that immobilizing the forearm for 2 weeks is useful to allow the skin around the pins to begin healing. This may help to prevent irritation of the pin sites. Alternatively, the wrist can be immobilized in dorsovolar splints. The splints are

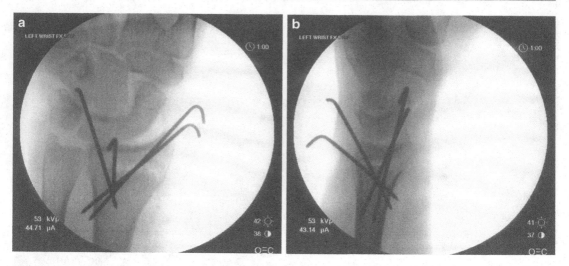

Fig. 15.11 (**a**, **b**) Final postoperative fluoroscopic scans after the K-wires are cut, bent, and left outside of the skin

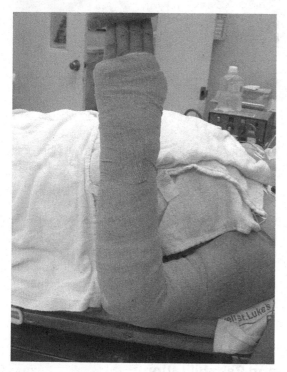

Fig. 15.12 The final dressing is placed consisting of a plaster sugar tong splint and overwrapped with Coban (3 M, St. Paul, MN)

secured with Coban (3 M, St. Paul, MN) or another self-adhering wrap with no tension (Fig. 15.12). After the initial 2 weeks of immobilization, the patient is seen back in the office for follow-up

radiographs. The wrist is then immobilized in a short arm cast if the DRUJ was stable at surgery or a long arm cast if the DRUJ was unstable and needed to be pinned during the surgery. Patients are then seen biweekly in order to obtain new radiographs. The cast is removed and the pin sites are examined only if the patient has complaints or if there is a concern about pin site infection or pin migration. Immobilization is usually continued for a total of 5–6 weeks postoperatively. We never immobilize a fracture of the distal radius for longer than 6 weeks. At that point, the cast is removed. If the fracture is nontender and if radiographs confirm maintenance of reduction and healing of the fracture, the K-wires are removed. The patient is referred to the hand therapist for a prefabricated wrist-resting splint, which is used for support and protection of the wrist for the 2 weeks after immobilization is discontinued. The patient removes the splint to work on range of motion exercise and scar massage. Range of motion can usually be regained within 4–6 weeks after the cast removal. Two weeks after immobilization is discontinued, gentle strengthening exercise with putty and a hand gripper is started. At 1-month after immobilization, light resistive exercises can be started using a 1- to 3-lb. dumbbell and progressing as the patient tolerates. At 3 months after fracture, they can resume all activities (Fig. 15.13a–c).

Fig. 15.13 (**a**) Pre-operative radiographs of a 46-year-old man with an unstable distal radius fracture. (**b**) Radiographs after minimally invasive fixation of the distal radius. (**c**) Final radiographs of the healed fracture 8 weeks after the initial injury

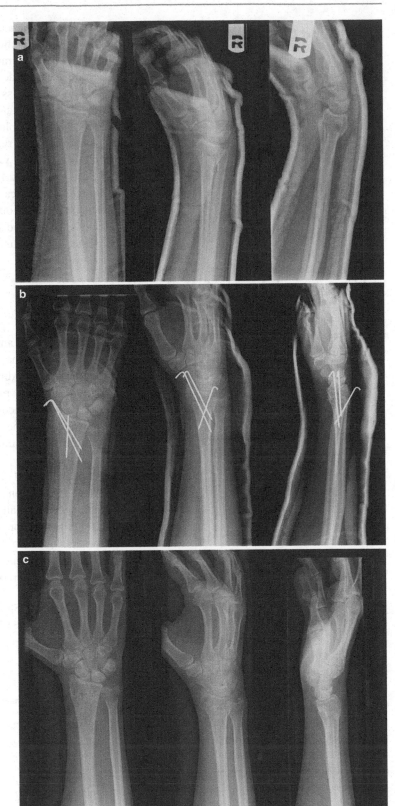

Results and Complications

Several recent prospective studies demonstrated the effectiveness of closed reduction and percutaneous pinning when the pins were placed in an orthogonal configuration [10, 11]. Follow-up studies in the past have shown variable results and have reported several instances of loss of reduction when fractures were solely pinned through the radial styloid [12–14].

In a prospective randomized study with 100 patients, Strohm et al. [15] compared two different procedures for pinning of distal radius fractures. One method of pinning was with two K-wires inserted at the styloid process as described by Willenegger and Guggenbuhl [2]. The technique to which it was compared was a modified Kapandji method as described by Fritz et al. [16] using two dorsal intrafocal pins and one radial styloid pin. They found the functional and radiographic outcomes to be significantly better in the patients who had intrafocal pinning and attributed the results, in part, to a shorter immobilization period in those patients. Complications were not significantly different between the groups. In total, 12 patients had nerve irritations that resolved after pin removal. Eight patients between the groups had wire migration, but none of the patients had tendon injury or rupture. One patient in each group developed carpal tunnel syndrome and one patient in each group developed reflex sympathetic dystrophy (RSD).

Minimally invasive fixation for distal radius fractures may also become a more desirable option than volar plating in amenable fractures as the long-term results are being reported. Rozental and Blazar [17] reported on 41 patients who underwent volar plating and who were followed for a minimum of 12 months. While all of the patients had good to excellent results, there was a 22% complication rate, of which 7% was hardware-related tendon irritation. Two patients had symptomatic subluxation of the flexor pollicis longus tendon over the plate and one patient experienced dorsal swelling and irritation caused by a prominent screw. Each patient had some improvement after hardware removal.

In our experience, we have been very satisfied with closed reduction and percutaneous pinning for unstable distal radius fractures. Complications are rare and include pin tract irritation and superficial infection, loss of reduction, and superficial radial nerve irritation. Fortunately, superficial radial nerve complaints have been minimal and resolve after pin removal, and we think this is directly related to visualization of the nerve during pin placement. It is also the authors' opinion that more complications from volar plating such as palmar cutaneous nerve injuries and flexor pollicis longus and EPL tendon ruptures will be reported in the future as the long-term results are reviewed.

Conclusion

Closed reduction and percutaneous pinning is a valuable technique for treating displaced and unstable distal radius fractures. The method is relatively simple, minimally invasive, and reliable. Good to excellent results can usually be achieved when the procedure is performed for the proper indications and biomechanically sound pin configuration is used. Complication rates have been low and manageable and have included pin tract infections and skin irritation. These problems can usually be treated effectively with oral antibiotics or pin removal. Injury to the superficial radial nerve is also a commonly reported complication that can be avoided with direct visualization of the nerve.

Acknowledgment Special thanks to Benjamin Chia, BA, for his assistance with preparation of the manuscript.

References

1. Lambotte A. *L'Intervention opératoire dans les fractures récentes et anciennes*. Paris: A. Maloine; 1907
2. Willenegger H, Guggenbuhl A. [Operative treatment of certain cases of distal radius fracture.]. *Helv Chir Acta*. 1959;26(2):81–94
3. Stein AH, Jr., Katz SF. Stabilization of comminuted fractures of the distal inch of the radius: percutaneous pinning. *Clin Orthop Relat Res*. May 1975;(108): 174–181

4. Clancey GJ. Percutaneous Kirschner-wire fixation of Colles fractures. A prospective study of thirty cases. *J Bone Joint Surg Am*. 1984;66(7):1008–1014

5. Fernandez DL, Geissler WB. Treatment of displaced articular fractures of the radius. *J Hand Surg (Am)*. 1991;16(3):375–384

6. Kapandji A. [Internal fixation by double intrafocal plate. Functional treatment of non articular fractures of the lower end of the radius (author's transl)]. *Ann Chir*. 1976;30(11–12):903–908

7. Kapandji A. [Intra-focal pinning of fractures of the distal end of the radius 10 years later]. *Ann Chir Main*. 1987;6(1):57–63

8. Naidu SH, Capo JT, Moulton M, Ciccone W, II, Radin A. Percutaneous pinning of distal radius fractures: a biomechanical study. *J Hand Surg (Am)*. 1997;22(2):252–257

9. Rogge RD, Adams BD, Goel VK. An analysis of bone stresses and fixation stability using a finite element model of simulated distal radius fractures. *J Hand Surg (Am)*. 2002;27(1):86–92

10. Harley BJ, Scharfenberger A, Beaupre LA, Jomha N, Weber DW. Augmented external fixation versus percutaneous pinning and casting for unstable fractures of the distal radius – a prospective randomized trial. *J Hand Surg (Am)*. 2004;29(5):815–824

11. Ludvigsen TC, Johansen S, Svenningsen S, Saetermo R. External fixation versus percutaneous pinning for unstable Colles' fracture. Equal outcome in a randomized study of 60 patients. *Acta Orthop Scand*. 1997;68(3):255–258

12. Habernek H, Weinstabl R, Fialka C, Schmid L. Unstable distal radius fractures treated by modified Kirschner wire pinning: anatomic considerations, technique, and results. *J Trauma*. 1994;36(1):83–88

13. Mah ET, Atkinson RN. Percutaneous Kirschner wire stabilisation following closed reduction of Colles' fractures. *J Hand Surg (Br)*. 1992;17(1):55–62

14. Munson GO, Gainor BJ. Percutaneous pinning of distal radius fractures. *J Trauma*. 1981;21(12):1032–1035

15. Strohm PC, Muller CA, Boll T, Pfister U. Two procedures for Kirschner wire osteosynthesis of distal radial fractures. A randomized trial. *J Bone Joint Surg Am*. 2004;86-A(12):2621–2628

16. Fritz T, Wersching D, Klavora R, Krieglstein C, Friedl W. Combined Kirschner wire fixation in the treatment of Colles fracture. A prospective, controlled trial. *Arch Orthop Trauma Surg*. 1999;119(3–4):171–178

17. Rozental TD, Blazar PE. Functional outcome and complications after volar plating for dorsally displaced, unstable fractures of the distal radius. *J Hand Surg (Am)*. 2006;31(3):359–365

Endoscopic and Minimally Invasive Carpal Tunnel and Trigger Finger Release

16

Mordechai Vigler and Steve K. Lee

Minimally Invasive Carpal Tunnel Release

Carpal tunnel syndrome (CTS) is the most common peripheral entrapment neuropathy [1, 2], with a lifetime incidence estimated at up to 10% [3], The pathophysiology of CTS is thought to be due to compression of the median nerve in the region of the carpal tunnel [4, 5]. When symptoms are recalcitrant to conservative management, surgical intervention is indicated. The goal of surgery is to decompress the median nerve in the carpal tunnel by transecting the deep transverse carpal ligament (TCL).

Surgical options include open or endoscopic division of the TCL. The gold standard of operative intervention has been the open carpal tunnel release (CTR), which was first popularized by Phalen et al. [6, 7]. In the open technique, this division is typically carried out through a longitudinal palmar incision. Direct vision allows a safe division of the palmar fascia, following which, the TCL is identified and divided longitudinally, with care taken to protect the underlying median nerve.

S.K. Lee (✉)
Division of Hand Surgery, Department of Orthopaedic
Surgery, The NYU Hospital for Joint Diseases,
New York, NY, USA

Department of Orthopaedic Surgery, The New York
University School of Medicine, New York, NY, USA

Hand Surgery Service, Bellevue Hospital Center,
New York, NY, USA
e-mail: steve.lee@nyumc.org

The most common complications after open procedure are hypertrophic or painful scars and pillar pain (pain in thenar or hypothenar eminences) [8, 9]. In an effort to decrease these complications, limited or short palmar incisions as well as endoscopic techniques have evolved, because these methods are thought to result in reduced morbidity versus more extensive approaches that violate all tissue levels over a greater distance [10, 11]. Proposed advantages of using a limited incision are decreased pillar tenderness and earlier return to work or avocational activities [12, 13]. According to several studies, endoscopic carpal tunnel release (ECTR) results in a notably more rapid return to work and daily activities, more rapid return of postoperative grip and pinch strengths, and less scar tenderness than open CTR [14–18].

The objective of this chapter is to describe the technical details of performance of the limited incision as well as two basic types of ECTR, namely the single-portal and two-portal techniques.

Limited Incision Carpal Tunnel Release

Security Clip Enclosed Carpal Tunnel Release System (Biomet Orthopedics, Inc.)

Indications

Patients whose CTS symptoms are unresponsive to conservative treatment after 2–3 months may be considered for operative release using the Security

G.R. Scuderi and A.J. Tria (eds.), *Minimally Invasive Surgery in Orthopedics: Upper Extremity Handbook*,
DOI 10.1007/978-1-4614-0673-0_16, © Springer Science+Business Media, LLC 2012

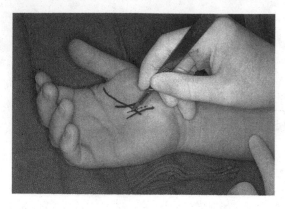

Fig. 16.1 Landmarks for the surgical incision. The incision is two thirds proximal and one third distal to the extended thenar muscle line and in line with the radial border of the ring finger (Courtesy of James W. Strickland, MD, Carmel, IN, with permission)

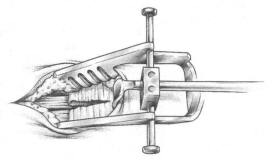

Fig. 16.2 Incision of the distal 1.5 cm of the transverse carpal ligament under direct vision. The specially designed, three-sided Biomet retractor facilitates exposure (Courtesy of Biomet Orthopedics Inc., Warsaw, IN, with permission)

Clip or standard open incision. Contraindications for the Security Clip include patients with a known palmar carpal canal mass, previous displaced wrist fracture, or any other condition that may have altered wrist morphology. A relative contraindication is a patient requiring concomitant open palmar flexor tenosynovectomy.

Surgical Technique

Local anesthesia is administered followed by pneumatic tourniquet inflation. The landmarks for the surgical incision are the distal border of the thenar muscles and the radial border of the ring finger. A line is drawn over the distal extent of the TCL in line with the longitudinal axis of the radial border of the ring finger. A second line is drawn diagonally from the thenar musculature. The point of intersection of the two lines approximates the most distal edge of the TCL (Fig. 16.1). The skin incision is approximately 1.5 cm in length. It is designed to be approximately two thirds proximal and one third distal to the extended thenar muscle line.

A self-retaining retractor is introduced (Holtzheimer or Biomet CTR retractor). A blunt, right angle proximal retractor is utilized to retract the soft tissue proximally exposing the distal edge of the TCL. The superficial palmar arterial arch is usually visualized and easily protected throughout the procedure. The distal aspect of the TCL is longitudinally incised for a distance of

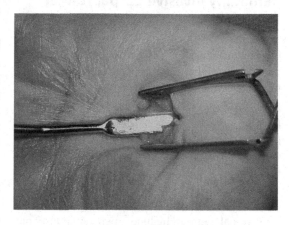

Fig. 16.3 The Blunt Single Pilot is passed beneath the transverse carpal ligament (Courtesy of James W. Strickland, MD, Carmel, IN, with permission)

1.5 cm using a scalpel under direct visualization (Fig. 16.2). The carpal tunnel contents can now be seen and protected throughout the remainder of the procedure.

Three instruments are used to clear any tissues adherent to the TCL. The first instrument, the Blunt Single Pilot, has a smooth edge and flat plane (Fig. 16.3). The purpose of the tool is to create a clear plane between the ligament and the underlying contents of the carpal tunnel. The pilot is placed just deep to the V-shaped notch created by incising the distal 1.5 cm of the TCL. The instrument is passed from distally to proximally, just deep to the TCL. The Pilot and all subsequent instruments must be directed slightly ulnarward to avoid injury to the radially vectored median nerve.

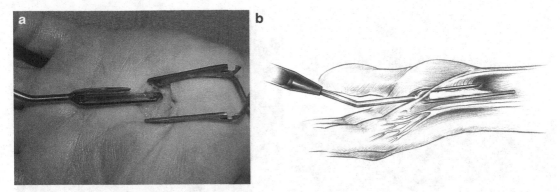

Fig. 16.4 (**a**) The Palmar Stripper with its long blunt lower skid and a short sharp upper skid. (Courtesy of James W. Strickland, MD, Carmel, IN, with permission) (**b**) Completed passage of the Palmar Stripper after it has prepared a channel through the dense palmar connective tissue (Courtesy of Biomet Orthopedics Inc., Warsaw, IN, with permission)

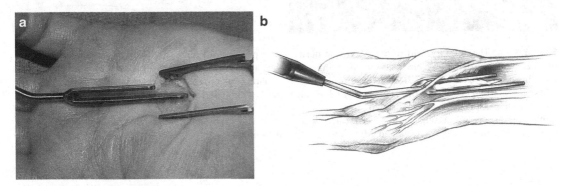

Fig. 16.5 (**a**) The Double Pilot with its blunt upper and lower skids. (Courtesy of James W. Strickland, MD, Carmel, IN, with permission) (**b**) Completed passage of the Double Pilot with the skids straddling the transverse carpal ligament (Courtesy of Biomet Orthopedics Inc., Warsaw, IN, with permission)

After removal of the pilot, the Palmar Stripper is placed into the wound. It is a double-sided instrument with a long blunt lower skid and a short sharp upper skid (Fig. 16.4a). The tool is designed to prepare a channel through the dense superficial fascia immediately palmar to the TCL. The distance between the two skids is 3 mm, approximating the thickness of the ligament at its distal third. This allows the instrument to straddle the ligament as it is passed from distally to proximally. Under direct visualization, the tool is inserted into the notch created by distal division of the ligament. The lower skid is placed deep to the TCL and passed proximally. The sharper shorter upper skid will pass palmar to the TCL. The stripper is passed until the blunt center post meets the edge of the V-shaped defect of the ligament (Fig. 16.4b).

After withdrawing the Palmar Stripper, the Double Pilot is introduced. The tool has long blunt upper and lower skids (Fig. 16.5a). There are no sharp edges on the skids that could injure surrounding anatomical structures (the Palmar Stripper is shorter and has a sharp upper skid). The Double Pilot enters the V-shaped notch created by the incision in the distal ligament. It straddles the ligament and is passed proximally to establish a pathway for the Security Clip. The Double Pilot is passed until the blunt center post is fully engaged against the distal edge of the ligament (Fig. 16.5b). It is critical that the instruments are passed sequentially using the same ulnar vector. All instruments

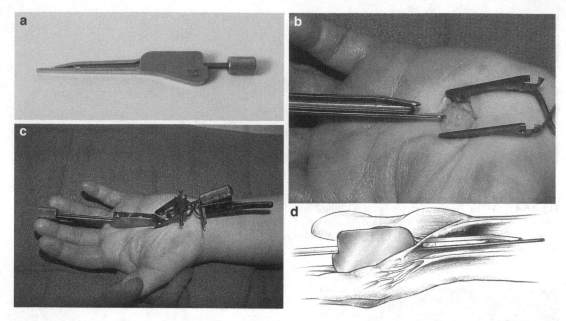

Fig. 16.6 (**a**) The Security Clip with the stylus in place (on the *right*). The disposable blade fits into the midline of the Clip device. (Courtesy of Biomet Orthopedics Inc., Warsaw, IN, with permission) (**b**) The Security Clip with the stylus in place is passed from distal to proximal, positioning the lower skid deep to the transverse carpal ligament. (Courtesy of James W. Strickland, MD, Carmel, IN, with permission) (**c**) As the Security Clip is fully seated, the stylus is automatically backed out of the device. (Courtesy of James W. Strickland, MD, Carmel, IN, with permission) (**d**) The Security Clip fully engaged with the TCL contained between the upper and lower skids (Courtesy of Biomet Orthopedics Inc., Warsaw, IN, with permission)

should be moistened prior to passage to provide better sliding characteristics. If some difficulty is encountered when passing the Double Pilot, it may be passed several times in a slightly different direction to be sure that there is an adequate channel for Security Clip passage.

The Security Clip is designed to protect the soft tissues on both the palmar and dorsal sides of the ligament. The lower skid has the same length as that of the Double Pilot. An upper skid is present, which converges on the lower skid terminally (Fig. 16.6a). The distance between the proximal end of the clip and the terminal closure of the upper skid is 3.5 cm. With this configuration, the Security Clip straddles the ligament, creating a closed system that is consistent with the usual morphology of the TCL. Prior to passing the Security Clip, a stylus is introduced into its central track, creating a 3-mm separation between the lower and upper skids (Fig. 16.6b). This facilitates positioning of the Security Clip into the

prepared channel across the ligament. As the assembly is advanced from distal to proximal across the TCL, the stylus will automatically be backed out by the edge of the ligament, and the distal tips of the instrument will close together on the ligament (Fig. 16.6c). When fully seated, the Security Clip will contain the entire TCL between its skids, and all other adjacent tissues will be safely out of harm's way (Fig. 16.6d).

With the Security Clip straddling the ligament, a disposable blade is inserted into the track of the device and passed from distally to proximally between the upper and lower skids (Fig. 16.7a). The blade is passed down the Security Clip, completely dividing the TCL. The upper and lower skids serve to protect the tissues dorsal and palmar to the ligament. Advancement of the blade continues until the disposable device fits flush with the Security Clip (Fig. 16.7b, c). Once the blade is fully seated, it is withdrawn. The Security Clip is then removed from the wound.

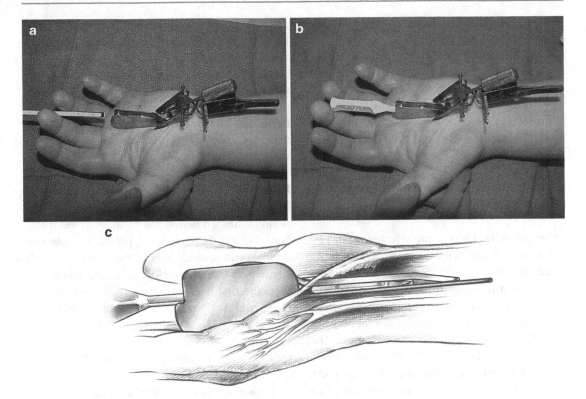

Fig. 16.7 (a) The disposable blade is positioned into the clip and passed distal to proximal between the upper and lower skids. (Courtesy of James W. Strickland, MD, Carmel, IN, with permission) (b) Advancement of the blade continues until it is fully seated within the Security Clip. (Courtesy of James W. Strickland, MD, Carmel, IN, with permission) (c) The Security Clip with the disposable blade fully seated within the device. The blade is positioned between the upper and lower skids protecting the surrounding tissue. The transverse carpal ligament has been transected at this point. (Courtesy of Biomet Orthopedics Inc., Warsaw, IN, with permission)

The soft tissues are carefully retracted proximally to confirm complete decompression of the TCL. A Freer elevator may also be used to confirm the interval between the transected edges of the TCL.

Endoscopic Carpal Tunnel Release

ECTR, introduced by Oksuto, et al. in 1989 [19, 20] has been promoted as an alternative to the open technique, largely to minimize the theoretical disadvantages of an incision through glabrous palmar skin and palmar fascia. There are two basic types of ECTR: single-portal and two-portal techniques [11, 14, 21–26]. Both techniques approach the carpal tunnel either proximally or proximally and distally from the limits of the thick region of the TCL. The endoscope permits constant visualization of the deep surface of the TCL, which is sharply divided through the same incision. The overlying palmar skin, subcutaneous fat, palmar fascia, and palmaris brevis muscle are preserved.

The overriding principle of ECTR is that it is of value in viewing and dividing the TCL but nothing else. It is not designed to explore the contents of the carpal tunnel. Patient selection, therefore, requires careful preoperative evaluation to exclude those individuals with pathology requiring direct inspection or surgical treatment of their carpal tunnel contents. Excluded are patients with rheumatoid synovitis, fracture, nonunion, congenital malformation of the hook of the hamate, calcific tendonitis, or deposits of gout or amyloid [27].

The techniques of ECTR are initially technically challenging and the surgeon should attend a formal instructional course prior to introduction of these techniques into clinical practice [28]. Additionally, one should be prepared to abort to the standard open technique if technical difficulties arise, such as inadequate views or difficulty in clearing tendinous structures from the field of view.

Endoscopic Carpal Tunnel Release (Two-Portal Technique)

Chow published his two-portal technique in 1989 and followed this with a report of his clinical results in 1990 [10, 14]. The original Chow technique was a transbursal technique in which the cannula system enters and exits the flexor tendon bursa. Since then, the modified Chow or extrabursal technique in which the bursa is not entered has been used. Nagle et al. [29] reviewed both techniques and concluded that the transbursal technique was associated with a higher complication rate and a higher rate of conversion to open CTR. Others have also concluded that the extrabursal technique is preferable [30].

Surgical Technique: Extrabursal Two-Portal Technique of ECTR (ECTRA System: Smith & Nephew)

As a prerequisite to surgery, it is necessary that the patient be able to hyperextend the wrist and fingers in order to perform this technique safely [31]. After adequate general anesthesia, regional block, or local anesthesia has been administered, the hand is prepared for surgery in the usual manner. A pneumatic tourniquet is inflated over the arm. A sterile skin marker is used to map landmarks and locate entry and exit portals (Fig. 16.8).

Entry Portal

The pisiform is palpated on the volar surface of the wrist within the flexor carpi ulnaris tendon at the distal wrist crease. A line from the proximal tip of the pisiform is drawn radially, approximately 1.0–1.5 cm in length. From this point,

a second line is drawn proximally 0.5 cm. A third line is then drawn from the proximal end of the second line radially 1.0 cm. This last line, which represents the entry portal incision, should be just ulnar to the palmaris longus tendon, if present (approximately at the level of the proximal wrist flexor crease) (Fig. 16.8). Average dimensions of these lines vary slightly, depending on the overall size of the hand.

Exit Portal

The patients thumb is placed in full abduction. A line is drawn across the palm from the distal border of the thumb to the approximate center of the palm. A second line is drawn from the web space between the middle and ring fingers to meet the first line, forming a right angle. A line bisecting this right angle is extended proximally 1.0 cm proximal from the vertex. This represents the exit portal (Fig. 16.8). Again, dimensions of these lines may vary slightly, depending on the overall size of the hand.

Creation of portals and placement of the cannula: A 1.0-cm transverse incision is made at the marked entry portal site, extending just through the skin. Subcutaneous tissue is bluntly dissected off the volar forearm fascia and retracted with Ragnell retractors (Fig. 16.9a). Care must be taken to avoid damage to the subcutaneous blood vessels. A transverse incision is then made through the fascia. The long blade of a Ragnell retractor is passed just beneath the fascia in a distal direction (Fig. 16.9b). The retractor should pass easily into the proximal aspect of the carpal tunnel. A Curved Dissector is passed into the carpal tunnel just under the TCL and above the carpal tunnel tenosynovium (Fig. 16.10a). It is important to keep the Curved Dissector pointed toward the planned exit portal to avoid inadvertent entry into Guyon's canal. The tenosynovium is often adherent to the TCL within the carpal tunnel. The tenosynovium should be bluntly dissected with the Curved Dissector off the carpal ligament and distal forearm fascia, from the proximal incision to the distal extent of the TCL. When the TCL is adequately prepared, drawing the Curved Dissector over the TCL should result in a type of "washboard" feeling.

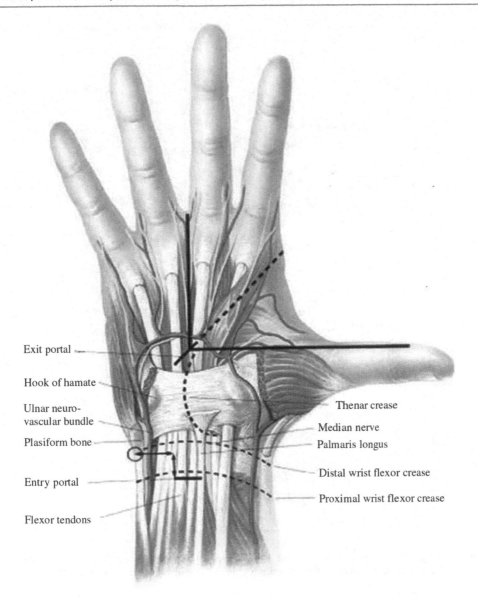

Exit portal

Hook of hamate

Ulnar neuro-
vascular bundle

Plasiform bone

Entry portal

Flexor tendons

Thenar crease

Median nerve

Palmaris longus

Distal wrist flexor crease

Proximal wrist flexor crease

Fig. 16.8 Entry and exit portals of the two-portal endoscopic carpal tunnel release technique (Courtesy of Smith & Nephew, Andover, MA, with permission)

The tip of the Curved Dissector should be palpated just distal to the TCL (Fig. 16.10b) and the location noted in relation to the planned distal incision. The Curved Dissector is then removed. A Slotted Cannula Assembly can now be guided into the space vacated by the Curved Dissector, following the route of entry created by its removal. The Slotted Cannula Assembly is advanced into the carpal tunnel on the underside

of the TCL just radial to the hook of the hamate, staying to the ulnar side of the carpal tunnel (Fig. 16.11).

The hand and Cannula Assembly are now moved as a unit and placed on the Hand Holder with the wrist and fingers in full hyperextension. The hyperextended hand is now strapped into the Hand Holder, following which, the Cannula Assembly is advanced along the underside of the

a

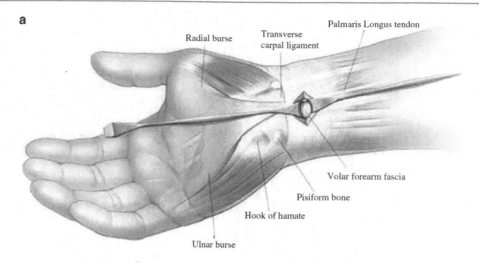

Palmaris Longus tendon

Transverse
carpal ligament

Radial burse

Volar forearm fascia

Pisiform bone

Hook of hamate

Ulnar burse

b

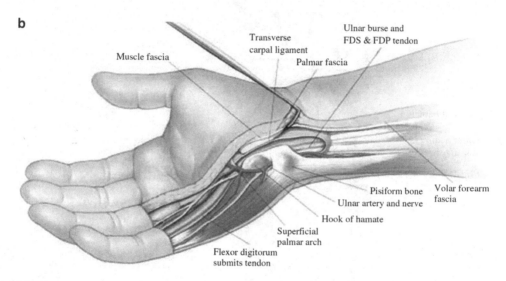

Ulnar burse and
FDS & FDP tendon

Transverse
carpal ligament

Muscle fascia

Palmar fascia

Pisiform bone

Volar forearm
fascia

Ulnar artery and nerve

Hook of hamate

Superficial
palmar arch

Flexor digitorum
submits tendon

Fig. 16.9 (a) Incision for the proximal entry portal. Retraction of subcutaneous tissue. (b) Long blade of the Ragnell retractor passed beneath palmar fascia in a distal direction (Courtesy of Smith & Nephew, Andover, MA, with permission)

TCL in line with the radial aspect of the ring finger until the tip of the Cannula Assembly can be easily palpated in the area of the mark for the distal incision (Fig. 16.12). The tension created by hyperextension, as well as the shape of the Cannula Assembly, causes the flexor tendons and other tissues to deflect from the pathway.

Care should be taken to avoid plunging the cannula assembly too deeply into the hand in a distal orientation. When the tip glides past the distal border of the TCL, it has entered the subcutaneous tissue. An incision is made just over the palpable Cannula Assembly tip. The incision is made only through the dermis and not into the subcutaneous tissue. The tip should exit proximally and superficially to the superficial palmar arch. The palmar skin and soft tissue is depressed using the Palmar Arch Suppressor, and the Cannula Assembly tip is then pushed into the receptacle of the Palmar Arch Suppressor (Fig. 16.13a).

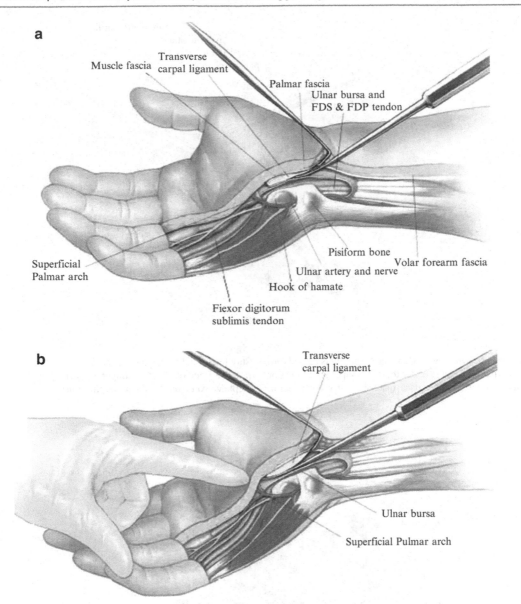

Fig. 16.10 (a) The Curved Dissector is passed into the carpal tunnel just under the TCL and above the carpal tunnel tenosynovium. (Courtesy of Smith & Nephew, Andover, MA, with permission) (b) Tip of the Curved Dissector palpated just distal to the TCL (Courtesy of Smith & Nephew, Andover, MA, with permission)

The obturator is now removed from the cannula. If positioned correctly, the Slotted Cannula should lie just below the TCL, superficial to the palmar arch and the branches of the median nerve (Fig. 16.13b). The slotted window of the cannula permits a safe cutting zone, isolating the TCL. The walls of the cannula guard vital tissues and delicate structures such as the median nerve and flexor tendons (Fig. 16.14).

Visualizing the TCL

The VideoEndoscope is inserted into the Slotted Cannula at the proximal portal. A thin bursal membrane may be seen above the Cannula's slotted

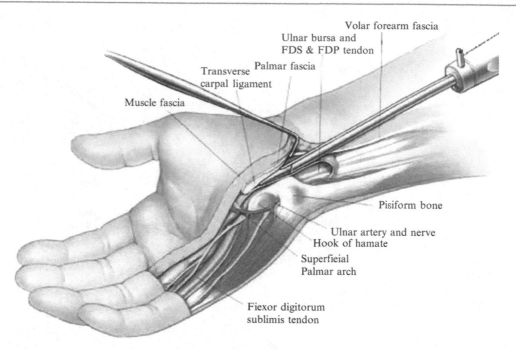

Fig. 16.11 The Slotted Cannula Assembly is passed into the carpal tunnel just under the TCL, superficial to flexor tenosynovium in the space made by Curved Dissector. Stay just radial to the hook of the hamate in line with the radial aspect of the ring finger (Courtesy of Smith & Nephew, Andover, MA, with permission)

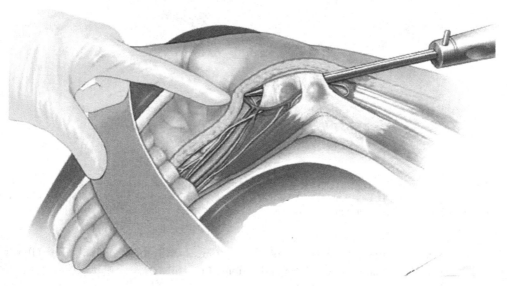

Fig. 16.12 The hand and wrist are positioned in hyperextension on the hand holder. The Slotted Cannula Assembly is advanced along the underside of the TCL in line with the radial aspect of the ring finger until the tip of the Cannula Assembly can be easily palpated in the area of the mark for the distal incision (Courtesy of Smith & Nephew, Andover, MA, with permission)

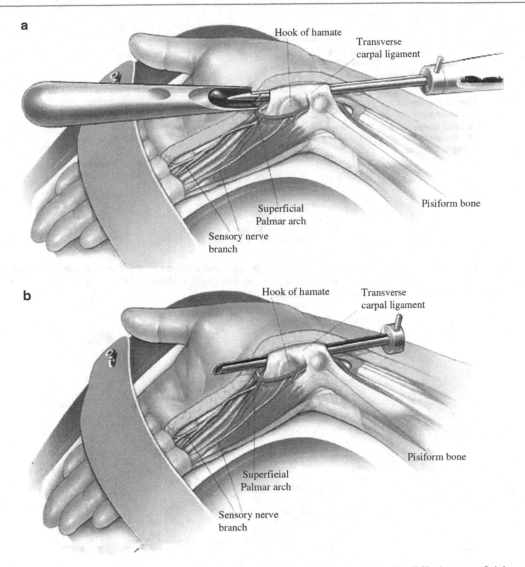

Fig. 16.13 (a) Palmar skin and soft tissue is depressed with the Palmar Arch Suppressor. The Slotted Cannula Assembly is pushed into the receptacle of Palmar Arch Suppressor. (b) Positioned correctly, the Slotted Cannula Assembly lies just below the TCL, but superficial to the palmar arch and branches of the median nerve (Courtesy of Smith & Nephew, Andover, MA, with permission)

opening. To gain access to the ligament, this portion of the bursa is dissected with a probe inserted through the Slotted Cannula's distal opening.

The TCL should now be identified by its fibers that run in a transverse direction. A white tissue with a swollen appearance, running longitudinally on the radial side of the opening, may also be seen. This is either the ulnar edge of the median nerve or the tendon sheath of the flexor tendons. It should be protected from injury.

The area is then probed in a distal to proximal direction until the entire TCL has been visualized. The TCL must be clearly seen with no other tissue visible between the ligament and the cannula. If difficulty in accessing the ligament is experienced, the VideoEndoscope should be removed. The TCL should be further prepared by the Curved Dissector. The Cannula Assembly should then be reinserted, the Obturator removed, and the VideoEndoscope reinserted.

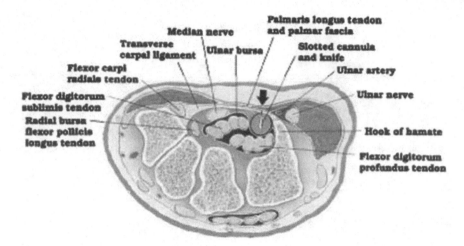

Fig. 16.14 Cross-section of the wrist. Slotted cannula and knife are shown in position within the carpal tunnel. The *arrow* indicates the site of TCL release. The cannula protects the contents of the carpal tunnel (Courtesy of Smith & Nephew, Andover, MA, with permission)

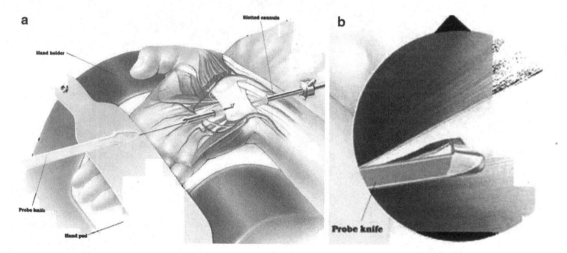

Fig. 16.15 (a) The Probe Knife, inserted in the distal portal, for forward cutting of the distal edge of the TCL. (Courtesy of Smith & Nephew, Andover, MA, with permission.) (b) The Probe Knife cutting the distal edge of the TCL, distally to proximally (Courtesy of Smith & Nephew, Andover, MA, with permission)

Release of the TCL

The Probe Knife, which permits forward cutting only, is inserted into the distal portal (Fig. 16.15a). The blunt surface of the knife can be used to probe proximally to distally along the ligament. The cutting edge is then used to release the distal edge of the ligament (Fig. 16.15b). The Triangle Knife is then inserted through the distal opening of the slotted cannula to the midsection of the TCL, and an upward cut is made (Fig. 16.16).

The Retrograde Knife is now positioned into the distal opening and its blunt tip is gently inserted through the incision made by the Triangle Knife. The cutting edge of the Retrograde Knife is drawn distally, making an incision that joins the previous two cuts, thereby completing the release of the distal aspect of the TCL (Fig. 16.17).

The VideoEndoscope is then moved from the proximal to the distal opening of the Slotted Cannula. The probe is inserted in the proximal

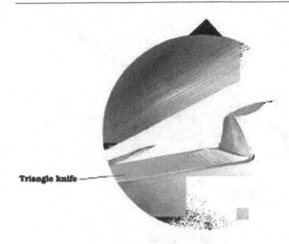

Fig. 16.16 The Triangle Knife allowing a controlled upward cut for incising the midsection of the TCL (Courtesy of Smith & Nephew, Andover, MA, with permission)

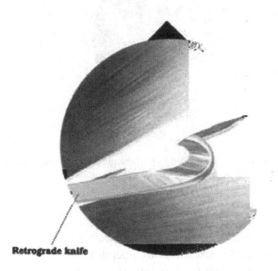

Fig. 16.17 The Retrograde Knife is drawn distally to join the previous two cuts, completing the distal release of the TCL (Courtesy of Smith & Nephew, Andover, MA, with permission)

opening. The Triangle Knife is used to initiate a longitudinal cut in the proximal fascia. The Probe Knife is then used to further extend the proximal cut. The Retrograde Knife is inserted into the midsection of the TCL from the proximal portal, then drawn proximally to join the previous cuts (Fig. 16.18). This completes the release of the TCL (Fig. 16.19).

Single-Portal Surgical Technique (MicroAire Surgical Instruments, LLC)

The first commercial version of the Hand Biomechanics Lab, Inc., device designed by Agee had a blade design that did not allow viewing of the point of penetration of the blade into the ligament. This limitation, combined with a problem related to blade elevation, led to a voluntary recall of the device. The blade assembly was redesigned to permit viewing of the point of entry of the blade into the ligament, and the device was reintroduced to the market in 1992. General or regional anesthesia is recommended, although the procedure can be done under local anesthesia [27]. A pneumatic tourniquet is inflated over the arm.

Skin Incision

In a typical patient with two or more wrist creases, an incision in a more distinct distal crease produces a better cosmetic result, whereas an incision in a more proximal crease is technically easier to use because of thinner subcutaneous fat. Of note, an incision in the more distal crease increases the possibility of inadvertently inserting the device into Guyon's canal. In addition, some patients have distal flexor creases that extend into the glabrous palmar skin on their ulnar extent. Wound in this glabrous skin should be avoided to prevent the possibility of a tender postoperative scar. The skin incision itself is made transversely between the adjacent borders of the flexor carpi radialis and flexor carpi ulnaris tendons (Fig. 16.20). It is centered over the palmaris longus, if it is present. The incision stops short of the subcutaneous tissues and their cutaneous nerves. A longitudinal spreading dissection is used to protect the subcutaneous nerves and expose the volar forearm fascia. The palmaris longus, if present, is retracted radially to protect the palmar cutaneous branch of the median nerve.

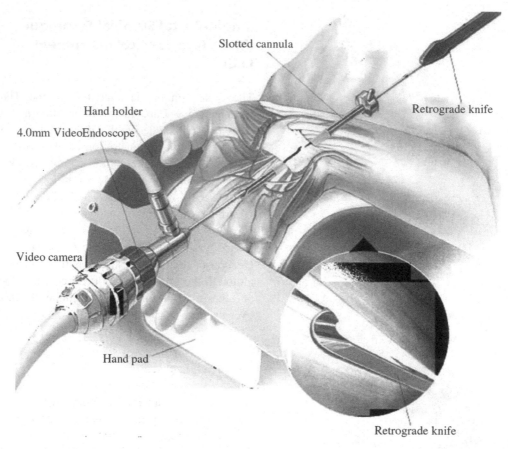

Slotted cannula

Hand holder

4.0mm VideoEndoscope

Retrograde knife

Video camera

Hand pad

Retrograde knife

Fig. 16.18 The VideoEndoscope in the distal portal. The Retrograde Knife is used to join the previously made distal and proximal cuts (Courtesy of Smith & Nephew, Andover, MA, with permission)

Critical surgical plane and release of TCL

A U-shaped, distally based flap of volar forearm fascia is incised and elevated (Fig. 16.21). The flexor tendon tenosynovium is then separated from the underside of the TCL by first the Synovium Elevator (Fig. 16.22) and then the Rounded Probe (Fig. 16.23). These tools should remain aligned with the ring finger, just radial to the hook of the hamate, and remain snugly apposed to the deep surface of the TCL. This positioning defines a path for the Blade Assembly.

With the wrist in slight extension, the Blade Assembly is inserted into the carpal tunnel and its viewing window is pressed snugly against the deep surface of the TCL (Fig. 16.24). Maintaining alignment with the ring finger, the blade assembly is advanced distally while hugging the hook

of the hamate to ensure an ulnar position. The distal advancement is to a depth of < 3.0 cm to avoid injury to the superficial palmar arch or the common digital nerve to the fourth web space. Proximal-to-distal passes are used to define the distal edge of the TCL [32]. Multiple techniques are used to define the distal end of the TCL: the video picture, ballottement, and light through the skin. With the Blade Assembly correctly positioned, the trigger is depressed to elevate the cutting blade and the Blade Assembly is withdrawn proximally, incising the ligament (Fig. 16.25). Several passes may be required when the TCL is very thick. A Ragnell retractor is used to protect the distal skin edge from laceration by the blade.

With the blade retracted, the Assembly is reinserted to inspect for completeness of ligament

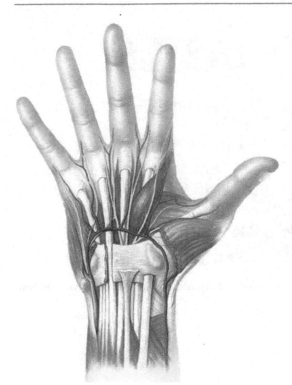

Fig. 16.19 Complete release of the TCL (Courtesy of Smith & Nephew, Andover, MA, with permission)

division. Completeness of ligament division is assessed by multiple techniques in addition to the video image. These techniques include palpation of the divided ligament with the Blade Assembly and the Rounded Probe, sensing the reduced pressure on the Blade Assembly when it is reinserted into the decompressed carpal tunnel, noting a more subcutaneous course of the Blade Assembly after ligament division, and direct inspection obtained by inserting one or two suitable right-angle retractors into the proximal end of the tunnel.

Endoscopic Assessment of the Completeness of Division of the Transverse Carpal Ligament

When viewed endoscopically, the partially divided ligament separates on its deep surface creating a V-shaped defect (Fig. 16.26). This is due to the superficial fibers of the TCL remaining intact. Subsequent cuts create a trapezoidal defect that is evident with complete ligament division when the two "halves" spring apart in radial and

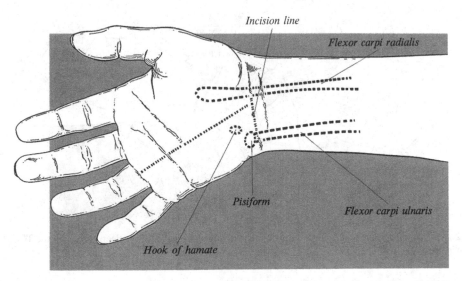

Fig. 16.20 Skin markings for the incision (Courtesy of MicroAire Surgical Instruments LLC, Charlottesville, VA, with permission)

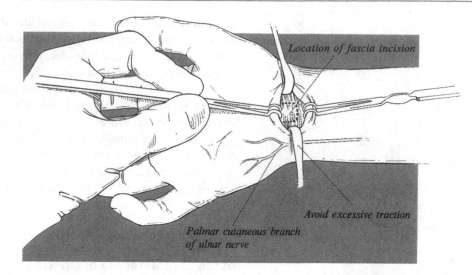

Location of fascia incision

Avoid excessive traction

*Palmar cutaneous branch
of ulnar nerve*

Fig. 16.21 U-shaped, distally based flap of forearm fascia is incised and elevated (Courtesy of MicroAire Surgical Instruments LLC, Charlottesville, VA, with permission)

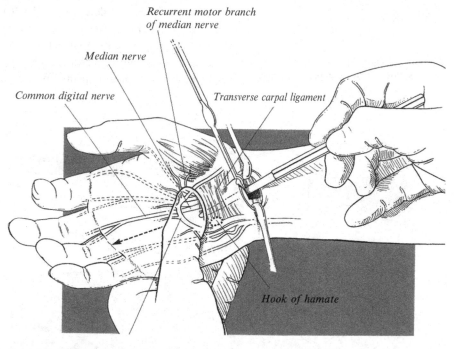

*Recurrent motor branch
of median nerve*

Median nerve

Common digital nerve

Transverse carpal ligament

Hook of hamate

Fig. 16.22 Synovium Elevator separating the flexor tendon tenosynovium off of the deep surface of the TCL (Courtesy of MicroAire Surgical Instruments LLC, Charlottesville, VA, with permission)

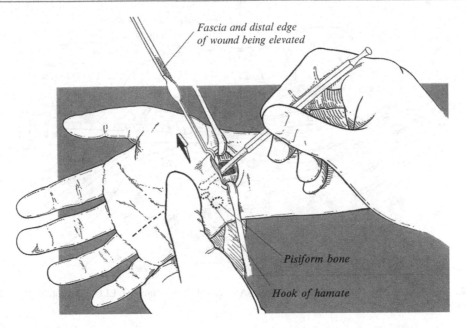

Fig. 16.23   The Rounded Probe is passed down the ulnar side of carpal tunnel to define a path for insertion of the Blade Assembly (Courtesy of MicroAire Surgical Instruments LLC, Charlottesville, VA, with permission)

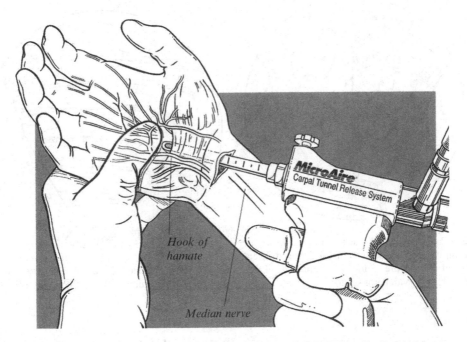

Fig. 16.24   Insertion of the Blade Assembly into the carpal tunnel (Courtesy of MicroAire Surgical Instruments LLC, Charlottesville, VA, with permission)

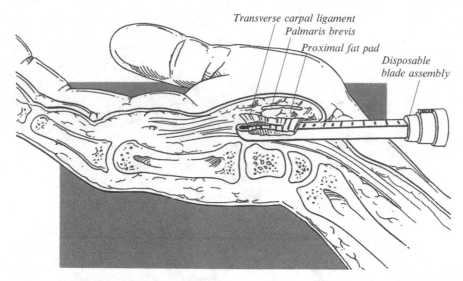

Transverse carpal ligament
Palmaris brevis
Proximal fat pad
Disposable
blade assembly

Fig. 16.25 Incision of the TCL (Courtesy of MicroAire Surgical Instruments LLC, Charlottesville, VA, with permission)

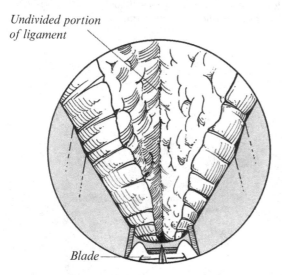

Undivided portion
of ligament

Blade

Fig. 16.26 Partially divided transverse carpal ligament, separated on its deep surface creating a V-shaped defect (Courtesy of MicroAire Surgical Instruments LLC, Charlottesville, VA, with permission)

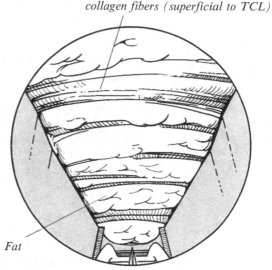

Remaining transvers bundles of
collagen fibers (superficial to TCL)

Fat

Fig. 16.27 Complete TCL division (Courtesy of Micro-Aire Surgical Instruments LLC, Charlottesville, VA, with permission)

ulnar directions (Fig. 16.27). The retracted fully cut ligament exposes transverse fibers of palmar fascia intermingled with globules of fat and muscle that can be forced to protrude by pressing on the overlying skin.

Release of Volar Forearm Fascia

TCL release is followed by palmar displacement of the carpal tunnel contents [33]. If the volar forearm fascia proximal to the carpal tunnel is

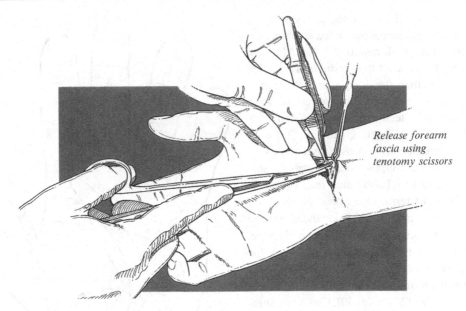

Release forearm fascia using tenotomy scissors

Fig. 16.28 Release of volar forearm fascia with tenotomy scissors (Courtesy of MicroAire Surgical Instruments LLC, Charlottesville, VA, with permission)

left intact, this palmar displacement occurs distal to the fascia, thereby possibly kinking the median nerve on the undivided edge of the fascia. This fascia should be released under direct vision with tenotomy scissors to ensure complete median nerve decompression (Fig. 16.28). The volar forearm fascia is divided for 2–3 cm in line with the ulnar aspect of the palmaris longus to avoid injury to the palmar cutaneous branch of the median nerve.

Minimally Invasive Trigger Finger Release

Trigger finger, or stenosing tenosynovitis of the thumb or finger flexor tendon, frequently occurs in adults. Triggering is produced by thickening (fibrocartilaginous metaplasia) of the fibrous sheath through which the tendon glides or by thickening of the tendon's normally thin synovial covering. Symptoms of triggering may also be produced by a tendon nodule [34] or by an enlarged tendon that locks the flexor tendon at the level of the first annular pulley (A1 pulley). Patients typically complain of pain, swelling, and

in some cases of having to grasp the digit with the other hand to extend the digit from its locked flexed position.

Numerous methods for treating trigger fingers have been developed. Nonsurgical treatments include extension splinting, administration of nonsteroidal anti-inflammatory drugs, and steroid injections. When nonoperative treatment fails, surgical release of the A1 pulley is indicated. Open release is typically performed via a small palmar incision under local anesthesia; the A1 pulley is completely visualized and incised. Although the success rate of open release is 97–100% with a recurrence rate of only 3% [35–38], complication rates of 7–28% have been described [35, 39]. These include digital nerve injury [39], infection [39], stiffness [40], weakness [39], scar tenderness [39], and bowstringing of the flexor tendons [41]. The open procedure requires an operative facility, and the surgical site requires wound care and can remain painful for up to 2 weeks [42].

Percutaneous release, using a fine tenotome, was first described by Lorthioir [43], who obtained good outcomes with no complications. A few decades later, Eastwood, et al. [44], reported the use of a needle tip instead of a tenotome and reported 94% excellent results. Several recent studies of the percutaneous release have also demonstrated favorable results [44–47]. Although percutaneous release for trigger digits is a quicker procedure [36] than the open approach, incomplete release or the need to convert to open release with this technique ranges from 0 to 11%[44, 48, 49]. Gilberts et al. [36, 38] concluded that percutaneous release was a quick procedure, was less painful, and obtained considerable better outcomes in rehabilitation than open surgery in the short term. One potential disadvantage is that it is a blind method; therefore, the approach can cause nerve or tendon damage. Nerve damage has not been reported with the percutaneous procedure, although it has been reported at the radial side of the thumb following open release [39, 42, 44, 48–50]. Cadaveric studies of percutaneous needle release have found superficial longitudinal lacerations along the flexor tendons in 88% of fingers and in all thumbs [45, 50]. This does not appear to have any significant consequences in most patients [46].

In this chapter we describe the technical details of the performance of the percutaneous needle and knife methods as well as the endoscopic method for trigger finger release.

Percutaneous Needle Release

Surgical Technique

Percutaneous release can be performed in the office setting. Local anesthetic is administered and the palmar base of the affected finger is prepared sterilely. The patient is asked to flex the affected digit actively. The surgeon then hyperextends the finger. This brings the flexor tendon sheath directly under the skin and allows the neurovascular bundles to displace to either side.

An 18-gauge needle is inserted at the proximal aspect of the A1 pulley. Care should be taken to stay centered over the flexor tendon sheath to avoid neurovascular structures and to enter the skin perpendicularly with the bevel of the needle parallel to the tendon. Alternatively, some investigators (and the authors' preferred method) have advocated inserting the needle slightly more distally in

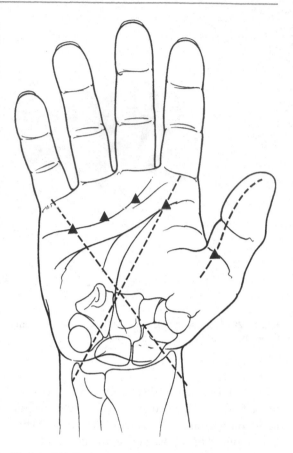

Fig. 16.29 Surface landmarks for percutaneous A1 pulley release. Index finger: at the proximal palmar crease at a line connecting the radial border of the pisiform and the center of the proximal digital crease of the index finger. Middle finger: at the distal palmar crease in the midaxis of the finger. Ring finger: at the distal palmar crease in the midaxis of the digit. Small finger: at the distal palmar crease at a line connecting the ulnar border of the scaphoid tubercle with the center of the proximal digital crease of the small finger. Thumb: at the proximal digital crease in the midaxis of the thumb (Courtesy of Biomet Orthopedics Inc., Warsaw, IN, with permission)

the middle of the pulley and then proceeding with release proximally and distally.

The proximal edge of the A1 pulley is located near the distal horizontal palmar crease for the small, ring, and middle fingers. For the index finger, it is located at the proximal horizontal palmar crease. Release of the ring and middle fingers is believed to be relatively safe. The oblique course of the flexor tendons and neurovascular structures to the index and small finger, however, pose a greater challenge. Wilhelmi et al. [51] (Fig. 16.29) described reliable landmarks for the small finger flexor tendon sheath in the area of the A1 pulley as lying underneath a line connecting the ulnar border of the scaphoid tubercle proximally to the center of the proximal digital crease distally. For the index finger, the landmarks were the radial border of the pisiform proximally and the midline of the proximal digital crease distally. By using these landmarks in a cadaver study, the A1 pulley was reliably transected. None of the digital nerves or arteries was transected. In the thumb, the intersection of the proximal thumb digital crease and a perpendicular line up the central axis of the palmar aspect of the thumb is the preferred insertion site.

The needle may be inserted into the tendon. This is confirmed by needle movement when the patient flexes and extends the distal phalanx. The needle is withdrawn slowly until this motion ceases. The needle tip is now in the A1 pulley. The A1 pulley is cut by moving the needle forward and back while advancing it in line with the longitudinal axis of the flexor tendon sheath. A grating sensation indicates the A1 pulley is being cut. Once the surgeon thinks the pulley has been released adequately, the needle is withdrawn and the patient is asked to flex and extend the digit to show relief from triggering.

Percutaneous Trigger Finger Knife (Biomet Orthopedics, Inc.)

Unlike percutaneous needle release, the Trigger Finger Knife is designed to avoid damage to the flexor tendons, avoiding possible complications of scarring and recurrent triggering.

Surgical Technique

Local anesthesia is used. Use a ruler to mark 1-cm-wide transverse lines, 1 cm and 2 cm proximal to the proximal finger crease. The approximate location of the A1 pulley is between these lines. The skin incision is made as a transverse line 3-mm wide and 3-cm proximal to the proximal finger crease (Figs. 16.30 and 16.31). A small pair of scissors may be used to gently spread the incision and palmar fascia if entrance is difficult.

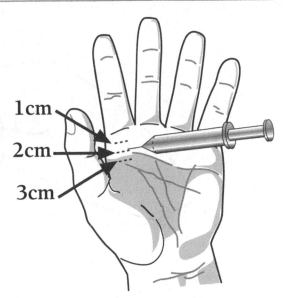

Fig. 16.30 Skin markings 1 cm, 2 cm, and 3 cm proximal to proximal finger crease. Local anesthesia is injected (Courtesy of Biomet Orthopedics Inc., Warsaw, IN, with permission)

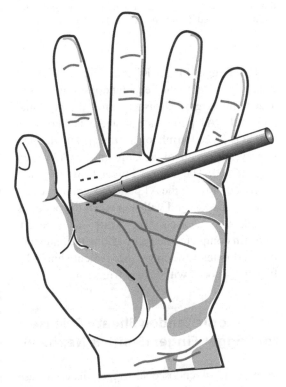

Fig. 16.31 The skin incision is at the most proximal of these marks (Courtesy of Biomet Orthopedics Inc., Warsaw, IN, with permission)

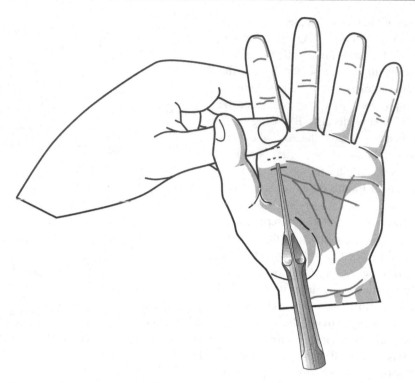

Fig. 16.32 The Trigger Finger Knife is inserted longitudinally, parallel to the flexor tendons. The surgeon's thumb is placed firmly on the distal skin marking to prevent passage of the knife into the A2 pulley (Courtesy of Biomet Orthopedics Inc., Warsaw, IN, with permission)

The Trigger Finger Knife is inserted longitudinally, parallel to the flexor tendons (Fig. 16.32). The knife is guided distally until the proximal end of the A1 pulley is palpated. The surgeon's thumb is placed firmly on the distal skin marking to prevent passage of the knife into the A2 pulley (Fig. 16.32). The Trigger Finger Knife is gently advanced through the A1 pulley. A grating sensation may be felt and will stop when the pulley is completely released. The knife is removed. Confirm complete release by asking the patient to flex and extend the finger. Movement should be free and smooth without any triggering.

Endoscopic Tendon Sheath Release for Trigger Finger (Smith & Nephew)

Proponents of endoscopic trigger finger release argue that it maximizes patient outcome by being a minimally invasive approach and yet releasing the A1 pulley under direct endoscopic visualization.

Surgical Technique

The procedure is performed under local anesthesia and the use of a pneumatic tourniquet. Two transverse incisions, each 2.5 mm in length, are made. The proximal incision is made 1 cm proximal to the proximal edge of the A1 pulley and the distal incision is located on the proximal palmar digital crease. The metacarpophalangeal joints are positioned in hyperextension. Separation of the flexor tendon and subcutaneous tissue is performed using a Curved, Blunt Dissector (Fig. 16.33). This is inserted proximally at the proximal incision site, and swept distally to create a channel.

The Window Cannula Assembly is inserted subcutaneously along the flexor tendon sheath from the proximal portal and advanced until it passes through the distal portal (Fig. 16.34). The obturator is then removed. A 2.7-mm, 30° Light Post Opposite Endoscope is passed into the proximal portal to confirm the extent of the stenosed

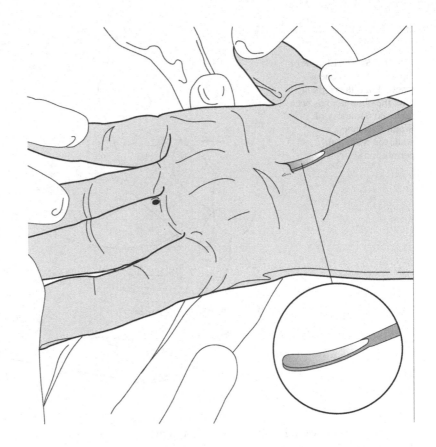

Fig. 16.33 A Curved Blunt Dissector is inserted distally to create a channel (Courtesy of Smith & Nephew, Andover, MA, with permission)

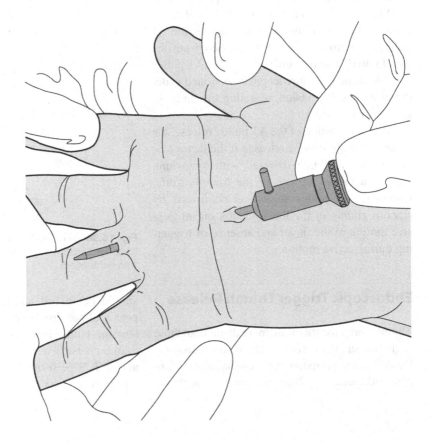

Fig. 16.34 The Window Cannula Assembly is inserted subcutaneously along the flexor tendon sheath from the proximal to distal portal (Courtesy of Smith & Nephew, Andover, MA, with permission)

Fig. 16.35 The Light Post Opposite Endoscope is inserted into the cannula after the obturator has been removed (Courtesy of Smith & Nephew, Andover, MA, with permission)

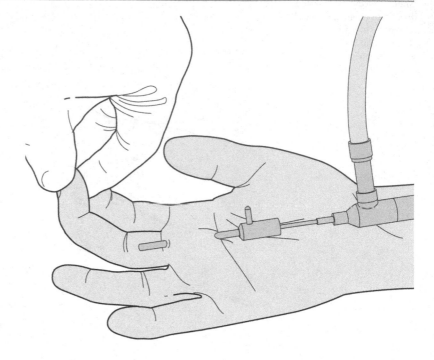

A1 pulley, and to examine the anatomy through the cannula window (Fig. 16.35). A probe can be used to palpate tissue, confirm anatomical structures, and pinpoint the proximal edge of the A1 pulley. A retrograde knife is inserted from the distal portal. The proximal edge of the A1 pulley is hooked and the entire length is sectioned under direct endoscopic vision, revealing the underlying flexor tendon.

After completion of the A1 pulley release, the synovial sheath may be released if the flexor tendon is longitudinally covered with synovium. This is achieved by use of the triangle knife. Complete A1 pulley release is confirmed by smooth gliding of the flexor tendon during passive motion of the finger and absence of triggering during active motion.

Endoscopic Trigger Thumb Release

Thumb portal locations are more distal than those in the fingers (Fig. 16.36). The distal incision is located at the midpoint between the interphalangeal and metacarpophalangeal joints. The thumb

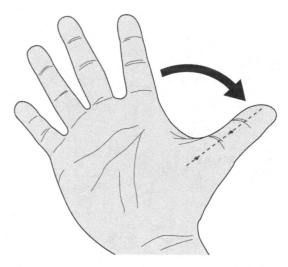

Fig. 16.36 Skin markings on the thumb for incision location (Courtesy of Smith & Nephew, Andover, MA, with permission)

should be in full abduction when making the proximal incision over the flexor pollicis longus tendon, 1 cm proximal to the proximal palmar thumb crease. The thumb procedure proceeds as above. It is performed in full abduction to avoid digital nerve injury.

References

1. Duncan K.H., et al., Treatment of carpal tunnel syndrome by members of the American Society for Surgery of the Hand: results of a questionnaire. J Hand Surg (Am), 1987 12(3): p. 384–91

2. Pfeffer, G.B., et al., The history of carpal tunnel syndrome. J Hand Surg (Br), 1988 13(1): p. 28–34

3. Stevens, J.C., et al., Carpal tunnel syndrome in Rochester, Minnesota, 1961 to 1980. Neurology, 1988 38(1): p. 134–8

4. Gelberman, R.H., et al., The carpal tunnel syndrome. A study of carpal canal pressures. J Bone Joint Surg Am, 1981 63(3): p. 380–3

5. Cobb, T.K., et al., The carpal tunnel as a compartment. An anatomic perspective. Orthop Rev, 1992 21(4): p. 451–3

6. Phalen, G.S., W.J. Gardner, and A.A. La Londe, Neuropathy of the median nerve due to compression beneath the transverse carpal ligament. J Bone Joint Surg Am, 1950 32A(1): p. 109–12

7. Phalen, G.S., The carpal-tunnel syndrome. Clinical evaluation of 598 hands. Clin Orthop Relat Res, 1972 83: p. 29–40

8. Semple, J.C. and A.O. Cargill, Carpal-tunnel syndrome. Results of surgical decompression. Lancet, 1969 1(7601): p. 918–9

9. Seradge, H. and E. Seradge, Piso-triquetral pain syndrome after carpal tunnel release. J Hand Surg (Am), 1989 14(5): p. 858–62

10. Chow, J.C., Endoscopic release of the carpal ligament: a new technique for carpal tunnel syndrome. Arthroscopy, 1989 5(1): p. 19–24

11. Agee, J.M., et al., Endoscopic release of the carpal tunnel: a randomized prospective multicenter study. J Hand Surg (Am), 1992 17(6): p. 987–95

12. Nathan, P.A., K.D. Meadows, and R.C. Keniston, Rehabilitation of carpal tunnel surgery patients using a short surgical incision and an early program of physical therapy. J Hand Surg (Am), 1993 18(6): p. 1044–50

13. Lee, W.P. and J.W. Strickland, Safe carpal tunnel release via a limited palmar incision. Plast Reconstr Surg, 1998 101(2): p. 418–24; discussion 425–6

14. Chow, J.C., Endoscopic release of the carpal ligament for carpal tunnel syndrome: 22-month clinical result. Arthroscopy, 1990 6(4): p. 288–96

15. Trumble, T.E., et al., Single-portal endoscopic carpal tunnel release compared with open release: a prospective, randomized trial. J Bone Joint Surg Am, 2002 84-A(7): p. 1107–15

16. Palmer, D.H., et al., Endoscopic carpal tunnel release: a comparison of two techniques with open release. Arthroscopy, 1993 9(5): p. 498–508

17. Brown, R.A., et al., Carpal tunnel release. A prospective, randomized assessment of open and endoscopic methods. J Bone Joint Surg Am, 1993 75(9): p. 1265–75

18. Kerr, C.D., M.E. Gittins, and D.R. Sybert, Endoscopic versus open carpal tunnel release: clinical results. Arthroscopy, 1994 10(3): p. 266–9

19. Okutsu, I., et al., Endoscopic management of carpal tunnel syndrome. Arthroscopy, 1989 5(1): p. 11–8

20. Okutsu, I., et al., Measurement of pressure in the carpal canal before and after endoscopic management of carpal tunnel syndrome. J Bone Joint Surg Am, 1989 71(5): p. 679–83

21. Adams, B.D., Endoscopic carpal tunnel release. J Am Acad Orthop Surg, 1994 2(3): p. 179–84

22. Bande, S., L. De Smet, and G. Fabry, The results of carpal tunnel release: open versus endoscopic technique. J Hand Surg (Br), 1994 19(1): p. 14–7

23. Brown, M.G., B. Keyser, and E.S. Rothenberg, Endoscopic carpal tunnel release. J Hand Surg (Am), 1992 17(6): p. 1009–11

24. Erdmann, M.W., Endoscopic carpal tunnel decompression. J Hand Surg (Br), 1994 19(1): p. 5–13

25. Feinstein, P.A., Endoscopic carpal tunnel release in a community-based series. J Hand Surg (Am), 1993 18(3): p. 451–4

26. Resnick, C.T. and B.W. Miller, Endoscopic carpal tunnel release using the subligamentous two-portal technique. Contemp Orthop, 1991 22(3): p. 269–77

27. Agee, J.M., H.R. McCarroll, and E.R. North, Endoscopic carpal tunnel release using the single proximal incision technique. Hand Clin, 1994 10(4): p. 647–59

28. Berger, R.A., Endoscopic carpal tunnel release. A current perspective. Hand Clin, 1994 10(4): p. 625–36

29. Nagle, D.J., et al., A multicenter prospective review of 640 endoscopic carpal tunnel releases using the transbursal and extrabursal chow techniques. Arthroscopy, 1996 12(2): p. 139–43

30. Seiler, J.G., III, et al., Endoscopic carpal tunnel release: an anatomic study of the two-incision method in human cadavers. J Hand Surg (Am), 1992 17(6): p. 996–1002

31. Chow, J.C., Endoscopic carpal tunnel release. Two-portal technique. Hand Clin, 1994 10(4): p. 637–46

32. Viegas, S.F., A. Pollard, and K. Kaminksi, Carpal arch alteration and related clinical status after endoscopic carpal tunnel release. J Hand Surg (Am), 1992 17(6): p. 1012–6

33. Richman, J.A., et al., Carpal tunnel syndrome: morphologic changes after release of the transverse carpal ligament. J Hand Surg (Am), 1989 14(5): p. 852–7

34. Hueston, J.T. and W.F. Wilson, The aetiology of trigger finger explained on the basis of intratendinous architecture. Hand, 1972 4(3): p. 257–60

35. Bonnici, A.V. and J.D. Spencer, A survey of 'trigger finger' in adults. J Hand Surg (Br), 1988 13(2): p. 202–3

36. Gilberts, E.C., et al., Prospective randomized trial of open versus percutaneous surgery for trigger digits. J Hand Surg (Am), 2001 26(3): p. 497–500

37. Benson, L.S. and A.J. Ptaszek, Injection versus surgery in the treatment of trigger finger. J Hand Surg (Am), 1997 **22**(1): p. 138–44

38. Gilberts, E.C. and J.C. Wereldsma, Long-term results of percutaneous and open surgery for trigger fingers and thumbs. Int Surg, 2002 **87**(1): p. 48–52

39. Thorpe AP, Results of surgery for trigger finger. J Hand Surg (Br), 1988 **13**(2): p. 199–201

40. Hodgkinson JP, et al. Retrospective study of 120 trigger digits treated surgically. J R Coll Surg Edinb, 1988 **33**(2): p. 88–90

41. Heithoff, S.J., L.H. Millender, and J. Helman, Bowstringing as a complication of trigger finger release. J Hand Surg (Am), 1988 **13**(4): p. 567–70

42. Fu, Y.C., et al., Revision of incompletely released trigger fingers by percutaneous release: results and complications. J Hand Surg (Am), 2006 **31**(8): p. 1288–91

43. Lorthioir, J., Jr., Surgical treatment of trigger-finger by a subcutaneous method. J Bone Joint Surg Am, 1958 **40-A**(4): p. 793–5

44. Eastwood, D.M., K.J. Gupta, and D.P. Johnson, Percutaneous release of the trigger finger: an office procedure. J Hand Surg (Am), 1992 **17**(1): p. 114–7

45. Bain, G.I. and N.A. Wallwork, Percutaneous A1 pulley release a clinical study. Hand Surg, 1999 **4**(1): p. 45–50

46. Blumberg, N., R. Arbel, and S. Dekel, Percutaneous release of trigger digits. J Hand Surg (Br), 2001 **26**(3): p. 256–7

47. Bara T, and T. Dorman, [Percutaneous trigger finger release]. Chir Narzadow Ruchu Ortop Pol, 2002 **67**(6): p. 613–7

48. Cihantimur, B., S. Akin, and M. Ozcan, Percutaneous treatment of trigger finger. 34 fingers followed 0.5–2 years. Acta Orthop Scand, 1998 **69**(2): p. 167–8

49. Patel, M.R. and V.J. Moradia, Percutaneous release of trigger digit with and without cortisone injection. J Hand Surg (Am), 1997 **22**(1): p. 150–5

50. Pope, D.F. and S.W. Wolfe, Safety and efficacy of percutaneous trigger finger release. J Hand Surg (Am), 1995 **20**(2): p. 280–3

51. Wilhelmi, B.J., et al., Safe treatment of trigger finger with longitudinal and transverse landmarks: an anatomic study of the border fingers for percutaneous release. Plast Reconstr Surg, 2003 **112**(4): p. 993–9

Round Table Discussion of Minimally Invasive Surgery Upper Extremity Cases

17

Evan L. Flatow, Bradford O. Parsons, and Leesa M. Galatz

Case 1

Dr. Flatow: This first case is a 55-year-old, right hand-dominant ex-police detective who was injured in a motor vehicle accident in 1978. We don't have the initial films of the shoulder fracture, but he was evidently treated with olecranon-pin traction for 5 weeks. We first saw him in 1988, when he was virtually ankylosed and had moderate pain. The pain became gradually worse over the ensuing 18 years, and is now unbearable (requiring narcotic pain medications). He is also frustrated with the stiffness: he has elevation of 90°, external rotation to negative 10°, and internal rotation with the hand reaching the buttocks posteriorly. Dr. Parsons, are there any joint-sparing options for this patient?

Dr. Parsons: Joint-sparing procedures such as arthroscopic capsular release and osteoplasty, or open debridement procedures, are options in cases of glenohumeral arthritis in patients with mild arthrosis without substantial articular deformity. These types of procedures can be very helpful in decreasing pain and improving motion in properly selected patients, especially patients who are too young or too physically active to undergo shoulder replacement. Gerry Williams has had

success with open debridement and a biological resurfacing of the glenoid with capsular tissue in carefully selected patients; younger, more active patients with primary glenohumeral osteoarthritis. However, once there are extensive arthritic changes, especially in posttraumatic arthritis where significant deformity exists, the success of these options is less predictable. In a patient such as this, I would offer two main options: continuing to live with the shoulder the way it is or considering replacement arthroplasty.

Dr. Flatow: I came to the same conclusion. With this degree of posttraumatic arthritis, I felt at least the humeral side required replacement. In some younger, more active patients, we have tried to avoid a polyethylene glenoid. Initially we tried just reaming the glenoid, but these have not done well, so we have moved to biological resurfacing, either with capsule or fascia as described by Burkhead, or with a meniscal allograft as described by Levine and Yamaguchi. However, the results are not always predictable, and this 55-year-old, though still active, was willing to modify his activities, and I felt a total replacement made sense.

Dr. Galatz: I agree – placing a glenoid offers the most reliable pain relief and does have proven longevity. However, there are technical challenges: the shaft malunion will make use of a traditional stemmed implant difficult.

Dr. Flatow: This was a problem. In mild malunions, variable anatomy prostheses have been advocated

E.L. Flatow (✉)
Peter & Leni May Department of Orthopaedic Surgery,
Mount Sinai Medical Center, New York, NY, USA
e-mail: evan.flatow@msnyuhealth.org

to allow adjusting the implant to the distorted anatomy. However, I have not seen the logic in turning a bone malunion into a metal one. I have preferred, when possible, to use a cutting guide to reset the prosthetic head to the tuberosity and shaft axis, ignoring the malunited head, and aiming to restore more normal mechanics. When the distortions are severe, as in this case, I have resorted to resurfacing replacements.

Dr. Galatz: The use of a resurfacing arthroplasty is an excellent choice in this situation. The use of this particular prosthesis is bone preserving. In this young patient, this offers the advantages of future reconstructive options.

Dr. Flatow: One big disadvantage of resurfacing is it is harder to expose the glenoid. In some cases, we have used the superior approach advocated by Copeland, **XX** but in this case we were able to perform releases, which allowed exposure through a deltopectoral approach. A minimally invasive axillary skin incision can often be used, although we used a standard deltopectoral in this case. This patient went on to excellent pain relief and substantial but not complete improvement in motion. His latest range of motion is as follows: he has elevation of 140°, external rotation to 40°, and internal rotation behind the back to L1 posteriorly.

Case 2

Dr. Flatow: This 57-year-old, right hand-dominant man fell more than 5 ft. off of a ladder, landing on his left shoulder. He is a retired police captain and an active golfer. There is no neurovascular deficit. He has ecchymoses in his arm and axilla. Dr. Galatz, you are one of the pioneers of percutaneous fixation of proximal humerus fractures – would these techniques be helpful here?

Dr. Galatz: This particular fracture is not a good one for percutaneous pinning. The reason is because of the comminution along the medial shaft and calcar area. Comminution in this area is a contraindication to percutaneous pin fixation, as it will lead to an unstable reduction.

Dr. Flatow: Dr. Parsons, would intramedullary devices such as locked rods be an option?

Dr. Parsons: Intramedullary rods are an option in some proximal humeral fractures. These implants, when used, are most successful when good bone and stout proximal fixation in the humeral head enables a stable construct. In a comminuted fracture such as this, especially when the greater tuberosity is involved, I would be concerned about blowing out the tuberosities during insertion of the rod, and about my proximal fixation once the rod was implanted. As a result, I don't think a rod is a great option for this patient.

Dr. Flatow: We elected a locking plate. It allowed us to secure the greater tuberosity with sutures to the plate holes, and to rigidly fix the head to the shaft.

Dr. Galatz: The use of a locking plate is an excellent choice as this affords stability needed for this difficult fracture.

Dr. Flatow: Some surgeons have advocated an extended superior deltoid-split approach, exposing and protecting the circumflex branch of the axillary nerve as needed. However, I have generally preferred the deltopectoral approach. He went on to excellent function and reasonable motion (Fig. 17.1a–c).

Case 3

Dr. Flatow: This 62-year-old, right hand-dominant woman presented 10 days after being struck by a car. She had rib fractures and this left proximal humerus fracture.

Dr. Galatz: This fracture is a valgus-impacted fracture configuration and is very amenable to percutaneous pin fixation. This is an excellent choice in this case. On the fluoroscopic views, the valgus deformity is not yet reduced, however, it is reduced in the final X-rays. Reduction of the valgus deformity by upward impaction using the described technique is critical for allowing the greater tuberosity to fall into anatomic position. The pins are best placed low along the surgical neck to engage the head.

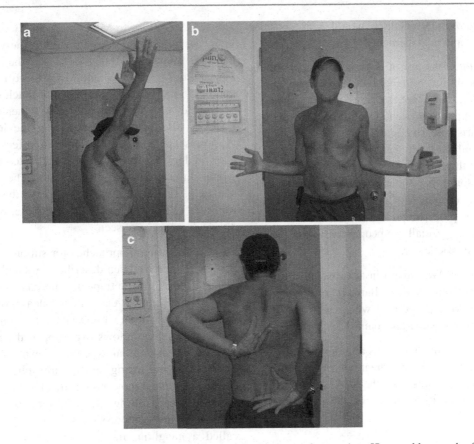

Fig. 17.1 (a–c) A locking plate was used to repair a proximal humerus fracture in a 57-year-old man who fell off a ladder. This patient went on to have to excellent function and reasonable motion

Case 4

Dr. Flatow: This is a 31-year-old, right hand-dominant woman who suffered a traumatic anterior right dislocation 6 years ago when she fell down a mountain. It took 6 h to get help and have the shoulder reduced. She has had four subsequent dislocations, all requiring manual reductions. The second also happened after a fall, but the last three were positional (e.g., reaching for a nightstand). On examination, she has classic anterior apprehension with abduction and external rotation, normal strength and motion, and mild generalized laxity (her elbows hyperextend to 12° of recurvatum and she can just approximate her thumbs to her forearms). Dr. Parsons – is she a candidate for a minimally invasive capsular procedure?

Dr. Parsons: The traditional surgical management of anterior glenohumeral instability has been an open labral repair with capsular shift if capsular laxity is apparent. Currently, many surgeons are performing arthroscopic repairs for instability with success, but there is still a role for open stabilization, especially in patients with glenoid bone loss or in patients with previous failed stabilization procedures. When indicated, these open procedures can be performed through a small, "minimally invasive" incision in the axillary skin crease that is very cosmetic and allows excellent exposure.

Dr. Flatow: Dr. Galatz, would you consider arthroscopic management?

Dr. Galatz: The use of arthroscopic stabilization for instability remains a controversial topic. However, there are several advantages of an arthroscopic approach. One is preserving subscapularis integrity and function. Even though subscapularis healing is reliable after instability surgery, there still is likely some compromise and this is somewhat substantiated in the literature. Another advantage of arthroscopy is the preservation of proprioceptive ability, which is easily disrupted, especially in people with some underlying intrinsic laxity.

Dr. Flatow: We did go in arthroscopically, and found not only a huge Bankart avulsion but a large SLAP tear, both of which we fixed along with some capsular tensioning.

Dr. Galatz: This highlights another advantage of arthroscopy: it allows treatment of concurrent pathology – in this case, the SLAP lesion, which can be very difficult to fix through an open approach.

Case 5

Dr. Flatow: This is an active 37-year-old, right hand-dominant man with right shoulder pain since an overuse incident working out with weights. Radiographs show an enchondroma (which had been biopsied) and no other abnormalities. He has marked external rotation weakness on examination, and an electromyogram (EMG) documenting suprascapular nerve dysfunction.

Dr. Parsons: External rotation weakness is usually due to one of two pathologic entities, a massive rotator cuff tear or suprascapular nerve palsy. In a young patient without history of trauma, the likelihood of a large rotator cuff tear is very low. Isolated suprascapular nerve palsy is often the result of a ganglion cyst in either the suprascapular or spinoglenoid notch. When I see patients with isolated external rotation weakness, I check both an magnetic resonance imaging scan (MRI)

and an EMG. Prior to MRI, we probably missed many cysts that were impinging on the nerve and causing weakness. When ordering the MRI, I make sure to tell the radiologist to go medial enough to include the suprascapular notch in the MRI field, or you may miss a cyst there. The EMG is also helpful in localizing the lesion. A suprascapular notch lesion will affect both supra and infra, while a spinoglenoid notch lesion would only effect the infraspinatus. The EMG also helps rule out a more global nerve dysfunction such as Parsonage–Turner syndrome, which, although rare, I have seen.

Dr. Flatow: Many approaches for suprascapular nerve release have been described. A small incision and a split of the trapezius directly over the suprascapular notch can allow release of the nerve at that location, while a small incision over the scapular spine allows exposure of the nerve from the suprascapular notch (by elevating a bit of trapezius and lifting up the supraspinatus) to below the spinoglenoid notch (by elevating a bit of deltoid and rolling the infraspinatus back). However, when compression is due to a cyst, also called a ganglion, most of us would use an arthroscopic approach.

Dr. Galatz: I agree. Spinoglenoid notch cysts are very easily treated arthroscopically. The cyst is the result of a SLAP lesion, which allows some synovial fluid to be compressed into the spinal glenoid notch area, putting pressure on the suprascapular nerve. If left alone, this can result in atrophy of infraspinatus primarily, but also of the supraspinatus if the cyst is higher, near the suprascapular notch. The cyst can be decompressed through an arthroscopic approach and the most important component of the repair is repair of the SLAP lesion. If this is not addressed then the source of the problem will not be eliminated.

Dr. Flatow: This is what we did, and the patient regained full external rotation strength at 6-month follow-up. He continues to have mild pain and weakness with overhead activities, but reports that he is much better than prior to surgery. He has returned to work on restricted duty.

Index